H A R L E Y   G O R D O N
Attorney at Law

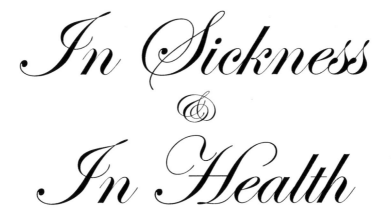

Your Sickness—Your Family's Health

How to Discuss and Create a Plan for Long-Term Care and the Consequences to Your Family and Finances if You Don't

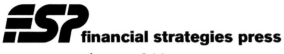

financial strategies press

phone   866-574-0031
fax   508-835-2280

Editing by Boris Levitin and Lisa Murphy

Proofreading by Lily Cox and Jennifer White

Design and layout by Boris Levitin, Luminophore, Boston

Printed in the United States of America by
Docuprint Express, West Bridgewater, Massachusetts

ISBN 0-9642896-0-1
Library of Congress Catalog Card Number: 94-61273

Acknowledgements

To my wife Susan, in memory of Ted, Phoebe, Eunice and Big.

*To my children, the best things that can happen in life —
Emily, Lily, Ben and Ian.*

To Ken and Daria Dolan. The success of this book is due in no small part to your belief in its author.

And finally, in memory of my parents Lewis & Eleanour Gordon. Your son misses you every day.

About the Author

Mr. Gordon is a founding member of the National Academy of Elder Law Attorneys, a non-profit organization that specializes in advocacy for the elderly. He has been voted as one of the 100 most influential people in long-term care by McKnight's Long-Term Care News. *His views on the consequences of not having a plan for long-term care have been featured in the national media, including* The Wall Street Journal, *the PBS documentary series* Frontline *and* The CBS Evening News. *His previous book,* How To Protect Life Savings From Catastrophic Illness, *was a best-seller.*

He has spoken at Million-Dollar Round Table's Top of the Table and national conferences including those of the Financial Planning Association, the National Association of Insurance and Financial Advisors, and the National Association of Health Underwriters. He was instrumental in creating the Certified In Long-Term Care (CLTC) designation (http://www.ltc-cltc.com), the country's only third-party designation dedicated to training financial-services professionals in assisting their clients' planning for long-term care.

Table of Contents

Chapter 1: Understanding the Consequences of Needing Long-Term Care 13

Why you need a long-term care plan 14

What is long-term care? 15

Long-term care is rarely nursing-home care 16

Who needs care: a look at statistics that don't mean much 18

Who provides the care 19

The cost of caring for you can be financially devastating to those you love 20

Providing care to you could make those you love as chronically ill as you 21

The consequences of not having a plan are real—and hurt 21

What is a plan for long-term care? 22

How to start a dialogue about long-term care with your family 23

If you're the one thinking about a plan 24

If you want to bring the subject up with your parents or relatives to whom you may have to provide care 24

Talking points 25

Wife discussing the subject with her husband 25

Daughter discussing the subject with her father 26

A niece discussing the subject with her uncle 27

Chapter 2: Types of Care: Everything You Need to Know ... 29

Levels of care 30

Custodial care 30

Activities of daily living (ADLs) 30

Cognitive impairment 31

Custodial care is most often given at home 31

Skilled care 32

Types of care are determined by the extent of the illness 32

Home care 33

Custodial care at home 33

Skilled care at home 33

Adult day care centers 33

Assisted-living facilities 34
Continuing Care Retirement Communities 35
Institutional care 36
    Hospitals 36
    Nursing homes 36

Chapter 3: The Best Long-Term Care Plan for You 37

Single, no children 39
Single with children 40
Married without children 42
Married with children 43
Second marriage with children 44
Divorced or widowed with children 46
Committed same-sex relationship 47

Chapter 4: Funding Your Plan 51

Paying for your plan 52
Self-funding 52
    Modest wealth: assets under $800,000 54
    Very comfortable: assets of $800,000–$2,000,000 55
    Wealthy: Assets in excess of $2,000,000 57
        Life insurance...58
        Home equity 59
Medicare 61
    Medicare *vs* Medicaid...61
    Medicare basics 61
    Medicare Part A 62
        Inpatient hospitalization 63
        Skilled nursing-home care 63
        Home care services 64
        Coverage.. 64
        "But my friend said Medicare paid for her Mom's home care"......66
    Medicare Part B 67
        Will Part B pay for custodial care at home?............68
    Medicare Part C: Medicare Advantage 68

Medicare Part D: The Prescription Drug Benefit 68
Veterans' benefits 69
Veterans Health Administration and long-term care 70
Eligibility..70
Will the VA pay for custodial care? 73
Benefits for long-term care based on financial eligibility 74
Funding is limited 75
The bottom line for veterans...75

Chapter 5: Medicaid **77**

What is Medicaid...79
Medicaid *vs* Medicare 79
Covered services...80
General medical services 80
Long-term care services 80
Medicaid and home health care 81
Qualifying for Medicaid..82
Medical eligibility 82
Financial eligibility...82
Assets..83
The look-back period 85
How a couple's assets are treated.......................................86
Community spouse resource allowance (CSRA) 86
Prenuptial agreements..87
Income...88
How an individual's income is treated 88
Cap states 88
Miller trusts...89
How a couple's income is treated...................................90
Minimum monthly maintenance needs allowance (MMMNA) 90
The Deficit Reduction Act of 2005 (DRA '05) 92
Planning for long-term care *vs* Medicaid planning...........................94
Life estates...99
Trusts...99
Revocable trusts 100

Irrevocable trusts 100

"Medicaid-friendly" annuities 101

Estate recovery 101

Illegal gifts 102

Still want to apply for Medicaid? 103

Medicaid planning in a crisis 103

Protecting a small business 104

If you have a disabled child: the supplemental-needs trust (SNT) 104

Protecting a primary residence 104

Choosing a lawyer 105

Interviewing a lawyer 106

Chapter 6: Understanding Long-Term Care Insurance 107

"Why do I need long-term care insurance?" 110

A brief history of long-term care insurance 115

How policies work 117

Basic policy parameters 117

Daily benefit (benefit level) 117

Benefit period 117

Pool of funds 117

How policies pay 118

Reimbursement 118

Indemnity 118

Cash benefit 119

Policy formats 119

Facility care only 119

Home health care only 120

Comprehensive care 120

Standard policy language 121

30-day free look 121

Guaranteed renewability 121

No prior hospitalization 121

Outlines of standard coverage 121

Specific exclusions 122

Unintentional-lapse provision 122

Benefit triggers...122

    Inability to perform activities of daily living 122

    Cognitive impairment..123

    Medical necessity...123

Elimination period...123

Bed reservation 124

Alternate plan of care 124

Home modification...124

Care coordination 124

Respite care 125

Waiver of premium 125

Optional policy provisions 125

Restoration of benefits 125

Survivorship option 126

Accelerated-payment (limited-pay, paid-up) option 126

Nonforfeiture 126

Return-of-premium option 127

Inflation protection 127

Tax-qualified long-term care insurance 127

Criteria of tax-qualified plans 128

Non-tax-qualified policies 129

Should you consider a non-tax-qualified policy? 129

Taxation of benefits of tax-qualified policies...130

Deducting the premiums on tax-qualified policies...130

Individual policyholders 130

    Eligible premium 131

    Non-self-employed individual policyholders 131

    Self-employed individuals (sole proprietors)..................................132

    Premiums paid for parents' policies 133

Partnerships..134

S corporations 135

Limited-liability companies (LLC)..136

Professional corporations (PC)...137

C corporations 137

State tax incentives 138

9

Employer-sponsored policies 138
    True group 138
    Affinity group 138
    Multi-life 139
Federal Long-Term Care Insurance Program 139
Long-Term Care Partnership programs 140
    Current protection methods.. 140
        California and Connecticut: dollar-for-dollar asset protection... 140
        New York: unlimited asset protection.................................... 141
        Indiana: hybrid asset protection 141
        Massachusetts: selective asset protection 141
    Partnership programs: advantages and disadvantages.................. 141
Paying for a long-term care policy.. 142
    Funding from an IRA 143
    Reverse mortgages (Home Equity Conversion Mortgages, HECMs) 143
    Life settlements 145
Children contributing to the cost... 145

Chapter 7: Buying the Right Long-Term Care Insurance Policy 147

When should you buy a long-term care insurance policy?................... 149
Step 1: Choosing the type of policy... 150
    Individual.. 151
    Joint policy.. 151
    Linked policy 151
    Life insurance with an accelerated benefit 152
Step 2: Choosing a daily benefit amount.. 152
Step 3: Choosing a benefit period.. 153
    If cost is an issue 154
    If cost is not an issue 154
    If there's a history of longevity or chronic illness in your family 154
    If you have a portfolio that is heavy in tax-qualified or low-cost-basis assets............ 154
Step 4: Choosing an elimination period.. 155
    Days of service 155
    Calendar... 156

Hybrid 156

Combination 157

Step 5: Choosing inflation protection 157

Compound inflation protection 158

When should you consider compound inflation protection? 159

Simple inflation protection 160

When should you consider simple inflation protection? 160

No inflation protection at all 161

When should you consider not buying inflation protection? 161

Guaranteed option to purchase inflation protection in the future 161

Inflation protection variations 162

Can I do without inflation protection? 162

Step 6: Choosing how the policy pays the benefit 163

Reimbursement 163

Indemnity 164

Cash benefit 165

Step 7: Choosing a benefit payout schedule 166

Daily payout: unused daily benefit is not transferable 167

Weekly payout: unused daily benefit is transferable to other days in the same
week 168

Monthly payout: maximizes flexibility 168

Additional options 169

Survivorship option 169

Accelerated-payment (limited-pay, paid-up) option 169

Nonforfeiture 170

Return-of-premium option 170

**Chapter 8: I Don't Qualify for Long-Term Care Insurance.
Now What? 171**

Paying for an uninsured spouse 172

Long-term care annuity 173

Medically underwritten single-premium immediate annuity (SPIA) 174

Chapter 9: Choosing a Long-Term Care Professional 177

Agents *vs* brokers 178

How to find a long-term care insurance specialist 179
    Word of mouth.. 179
    The Internet 179
Questions to ask your long-term care insurance professional 180
    Training 180
    Professional designation 180

Appendix A: State Medicaid Worksheet 183

Appendix B: Medicaid Life Expectancy Tables 189

Appendix C: State Tax Incentives 191

Index 193

Understanding the Consequences of Needing Long-Term Care

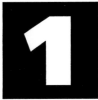

Why you need a long-term care plan 14

What is long-term care? 15

    Long-term care is rarely nursing-home care 16

    Who needs care: a look at statistics that don't mean much 18

    Who provides the care 19

    The cost of caring for you can be financially devastating to those you love 20

    Providing care to you could make those you love as chronically ill as you 21

    The consequences of not having a plan are real—and hurt 21

What is a plan for long-term care? 22

    How to start a dialogue about long-term care with your family 23

    If you're the one thinking about a plan 24

    If you want to bring the subject up with your parents or relatives to whom you may

        have to provide care 24

        Talking points 25

            Wife discussing the subject with her husband 25

            Daughter discussing the subject with her father 26

            A niece discussing the subject with her uncle 27

▼ N O T E S   **Why you need a long-term care plan**

My dad, Lew Gordon, had an outlook on life that was shaped by the Depression and tempered by service in World War II. After the war, he met Eleanour Shapiro at Winthrop Beach in Massachusetts and married her two years later. They set out to do what most twenty-five-year-old married couples did in that day: start a family.

My parents had five children. They raised us in a lifestyle that they never knew in their childhoods. My dad went to work for his father at Gordon Furniture in Arlington, Mass., and the two built a successful business.

As I grew up, I never thought of my dad as old. He was a successful man with youthful features and an athletic build. He was always busy and productive—always doing something.

I'll never forget the moment I looked at him and saw an old man. My parents had just returned from eight months in Florida. My father was sitting at the kitchen table, slumped over a cane and barely able to lift his head. I was stunned. Somehow my father had "suddenly" gotten old.

That day changed my life forever. I realized then that my father, who had dedicated his life to caring for his children, would soon need to be taken care of by his children.

That realization made me think of the paradox of long-term care: the person needing it is not the problem; one way or the other he or she will be taken care of. Rather, it is the impact providing care will have on his family. Put simply, your failure to consider the consequences of needing long-term care risks your family's physical and emotional wellbeing. It also jeopardizes your ability to fund a post-retirement lifestyle and keep commitments to those you love and the community because you will likely have to reallocate income to pay for care.

This need for a plan for long-term care is created by the historical confluence of three simple irrefutable truths:

1. People are living longer.

2. Living a long life creates the likelihood of needing care over a period of time.

3. Rapid advances in treating these illnesses make it inevitable that people will live longer with them.

Now, you may not believe that you will live a long life or that you may eventually need care, and you may be right. But if you're wrong, the failure to consider what providing care to you could do to those you love will have catastrophic consequences.

To put it directly: this is a book not about you, but about those who care about you. It is a study not of risk, but of consequences.

The good news is that these consequences can be avoided by creating a plan for long-term care. A proper plan will allow you to receive the majority of care, if needed, at home, while minimizing the impact providing it will have on your spouse, children or others you love. It will also protect your retirement portfolio so it can be used for the purpose always intended, paying for a post-retirement lifestyle and keeping promises to your family and community.

What is long-term care?

The term *long-term care* generally refers to assistance a chronically ill person needs to get through the day. It can include help with very basic housekeeping chores, such as cooking meals, paying bills, and using the telephone. It almost always

▼ N O T E S involves assistance with the most personal aspects of some-one's life, such as help with personal hygiene, dressing, eating and transferring from one place to another.

The U.S. Senate Special Committee on Aging explains how long-term care differs from other types of health care:

> *The goal of long-term care is not to cure an illness, but to allow an individual to attain and maintain an optimal level of function-ing...Long-term care encompasses a wide array of medical, social, personal, and supportive and specialized housing services needed by individuals who have lost some capacity for self-care because of a chronic illness or disabling condition.*[1]

Most long-term care is provided at home. The goal of home care is to allow the individual to remain independent in the community for as long as possible. As a sickness or disability progresses, home care may become more intensive, adult day care may be needed or a move into an assisted-living facility may become necessary.

Long-term care is rarely nursing-home care

Wherever you turn for information about long-term care, you invariably read about nursing-home care and what the chance is of needing it. The reality, however, is that it is unlikely you will need care in a facility: between the ages of 65 and 85, a weighted average of approximately only 3% of people will end their lives in one. Past the age of 85, the percentage rises to just under 19%.[2] It was never 43% as suggested by some

---

1 U.S. Senate, Special Committee on Aging, *Developments in Aging: 1997 and 1998,* Volume 1, Report 106-229, 2000
http://frwebgate.access.gpo.gov/cgi-bin/getdoc.cgi?dbname=106_cong_reports&docid=f:sr229v1.106

2 U.S. Administration on Aging & AARP, Washington, DC: *A Profile of Older Americans,* 2002

marketers of long-term care insurance. That survey stated that 43% of the population over 65 may spend some time in a facility, which could be as little as a day or week.

In fact, people don't go to nursing homes when they should. They go when the caregiver becomes so ill that the children have to take the decision away from her or him.

What they see is the person providing the care beginning to fail physically and emotionally because of the stress associated with providing it. Even then, the decision is almost impossible to make because the family never anticipated it:

> *"The tears have finally arrived. I feel like my dad is being locked away, and I'm powerless to do anything about it. I guess I must be in denial, but I can't imagine him living in a nursing home. It's just so heart wrenching.*
>
> *As I was leaving the nursing home he came out of his room and followed me to the elevator. He asked if he could go home with me. I had to lie and tell him he could after a while, but not now. I'm just so sad. I don't know what to do. I just can't live with the decisions I have made. Whatever I do is wrong."*
>
> *A Massachusetts attorney reflecting on placing her father in a nursing home*

Clients have told me that over the years:

> *"Whatever I do is wrong. If I keep my father home one more minute I may end up needing care. But if I place my dad in a nursing home I won't be able to live with the guilt."*

▼ NOTES **Who needs care: a look at statistics that don't mean much**

Here are some facts and numbers that simply confirm what you already know: People are living healthier, and as a result, they're living longer. Today, there are almost 40% more Americans age 85 and older than there were in 1900.[3] One out of five people who are 65 and older have self-care or mobility limitations, and one out of nine suffers from cognitive or mental limitations.[4]

So why are these statistics of no value? Reasonable people must believe that the worst in life will happen to…the next fellow. Like you, I am absolutely convinced that I won't get Alzheimer's, regardless of statistics saying I may. If I don't think I'll get sick, there are no consequences to my family or finances, so why plan?

In other words, the risk of something happening to me isn't going to motivate me to plan for it. On the other hand if I understood that, were I diagnosed with dementia, the consequences to my family and retirement portfolio could be severe, I would likely take action to protect both.

Very simply, the more severe the consequences of an event are to a person's family, the less the risk of the event happening to him has to be.

Two examples:

- Statistically there is only about a 2% chance of dying during one's working years. Why then do millions of people buy term life insurance? One word: conse-

---

3 U.S. Administration on Aging
   http://www.aoa.gov/prof/Statistics/profile/2004/2.asp

4 AARP., Washington, DC: *AARP Across the States: Profiles of Long-Term Care,* 2004
   http://assets.aarp.org/rgcenter/post-import/d18202_2004_ats.pdf

quences. For people who love their family, a 2% chance of dying is too high.

- Like most people, you may believe you are at little or no risk of needing care over a period of years, and you likely are correct: the worst will happen to someone else. But what if you are wrong? The answer is summed up in one word: consequences. The consequences are to your family and friends who will have no choice but to take care of you. Then there are the consequences to their financial well-being because your retirement portfolio will have to be reallocated to pay for care.

If you truly understand what I have just said, then any chance of needing care, even near zero, is now too high.

Who provides the care

Here is a sobering look at what providing care does to those you love:[5]

Spouses provide little care: In only 6% of long-term care cases in which the patient is fifty years old or older does the spouse play the role of caregiver.

Families provide care: In 83% of cases surveyed caregivers are family members of the sick or disabled person. Most caregivers are middle-aged women who care for one or more of their aging parents. They're often the oldest daughters, hold full-time jobs and have their own immediate families.

Caregivers tend to fall between the ages of 35 and 64, which means many are members of the sandwich genera-

---

5 National Alliance for Caregiving, Bethesda, MD and AARP., Washington, DC: *Caregiving in the U.S.,* 2004
http://www.caregiving.org/data/04finalreport.pdf

▼ N O T E S   tion—they're in the midst of raising their own children while caring for older relatives. A large number of these caregivers are also employed. 48% work full time, while 11% have part-time jobs. Nearly half of caregivers say they spend more than eight hours a week providing care. One in four spends nine to twenty hours a week and almost one in five provides forty or more hours of care per week—a full-time job in itself.

The average caregiver can spend more than four years of her or his life providing care for an ailing loved one.

The cost of caring for you can be financially devastating to those you love

Working caregivers face unique challenges. Many find themselves leaving work early on a regular basis or taking unpaid leave to dedicate the time needed to provide appropriate care for a sick family member.

These challenges have particularly adverse financial affects on female caregivers, because women spend an average of twelve years out of the workforce raising children and providing long-term care to aging relatives. That's twelve fewer years they're not earning a paycheck (an average loss of $566,000), which results in decreased Social Security retirement benefits (an average loss of $25,500) and retirement savings down the road.[6]

There's also the cost of commuting. Some long-distance caregivers (those who live more than one hour from the person to whom they provide care) spend about $400 a month on travel

---

6   Metropolitan Life Insurance Company, MetLife Mature Market Institute, New York: *The Metlife Juggling Act Study: Balancing Caregiving with Work and the Costs Involved,* 1999.

and out-of-pocket expenses in order to execute their caregiving responsibilities.[7]

Providing care to you could make those you love as chronically ill as you

Beyond the time commitment and financial repercussions, providing long-term care can also have a negative impact on the physical wellbeing of an otherwise healthy caregiver.

While caring for someone you love is honorable and can be a rewarding experience, it can also cause serious mental and physical stress. In fact, caregivers often suffer from increased blood pressure,[8] increased stress, and, commonly, depression.[9]

The consequences of not having a plan are real—and hurt

Every statistic I just mentioned was confirmed in my daily practice as an elder-law attorney. The person who came to see me wasn't the one who needed care. It was his spouse, children and other family members who were actively providing it.

While these families came from diverse backgrounds, they shared the same story. The person needing care:

- rarely expected to live a long life.

---

7   National Alliance for Caregiving, Bethesda, MD and AARP., Washington, DC: *Caregiving in the U.S.,* 2004
    http://www.caregiving.org/data/04finalreport.pdf

8   Cannuscio, C.C., J. Jones, I. Kawachi, G.A. Colditz, L. Berkman and E. Rimm: Reverberation of Family Illness: A Longitudinal Assessment of Informal Caregiver and Mental Health Status in the Nurses' Health Study, *American Journal of Public Health* 92:305-1311, 2002

9   Schulz, R., A.T. O-Brien, J. Bookwals and K. Fleissner, Psychiatric and Physical Morbidity Effects of Dementia Caregiving: Prevalance, Correlates, and Causes, *The Gerontologist* 35:771-791, 1995

- never thought he would need long-term care if he did live a long life.

- had no idea of what providing care to him would do to his family until it was too late.

Then there were the financial consequences. Many clients told me that prior to the illness their parents lived a modest but independent life. Paying for care, however, forced them to reallocate their retirement portfolio and income. The lifestyle of most was destroyed, and many had to turn to their children for financial help.

The consequences were never put more simply and elegantly than in a statement made by a caregiver in the PBS documentary *And Thou Shalt Honor*. Asked to reflect on what taking care of her husband, who suffered from Alzheimer's disease, was doing to her, she stated:

> *"When I got married, I never understood what 'in sickness and in health' meant. Now I do:*
>
> *His sickness, my health.*
>
> *For it to be easy for me, it would have to be over for him, and that's unacceptable.*
>
> *I often wonder: Will there be anything left of me, will there be anything left for me."*

This man has Alzheimer's; his family suffers from it.

What is a plan for long-term care?

By now you should have a clear idea of what providing care to you does to those you love. Creating a plan for long-term care, however, can protect your family and finances from these consequences.

The plan is composed of two elements:

1. Predetermined guidelines that define how and where an individual wants to receive long-term care, if necessary; and

2. A funding mechanism to pay for the care.

How to start a dialogue about long-term care with your family

Before starting the discussion, the first step is to ensure that the family understands the concept of risk versus consequences. Every one of my clients told me that their parents never understood the consequences needing care would have to their family and finances. You must understand that even though you deeply believe that you may not live a long life and need care, if you do need it, the consequences to your family and finances could be catastrophic. From this perspective, any risk of needing care, even if you think it is virtually zero, is now too high.

The second step is to begin a conversation within your family about what might happen if you or someone you love needs care over a period of time. Nobody wants to think about getting sick, being dependent on other people or moving into a facility, but the discomfort of talking about the subject is clearly outweighed by the consequences of not having that conversation.

▼ NOTES   The ideal time to consider the following discussion is between ages 50 and 65, for two reasons:

1. You are far more likely to understand what long-term care can do to a family, because many of your friends are experiencing it.

2. If a plan for long-term care makes sense, you are more likely to qualify for long-term care insurance medically.

If you're the one thinking about a plan

Start with your spouse. Be sure to put aside enough time to explain your concerns. Once you have the basics of a plan, consider discussing it with your children. You want to leave them with the impression that you and your spouse are in control of your care and where it will be given. This takes a tremendous burden off of children in their thirties and fourties who are beginning to worry about their parents' growing old. Review the talking points below for ideas on how to conduct the conversation.

If you want to bring the subject up with your parents or relatives to whom you may have to provide care

The most important thing to keep in mind is that the discussion must focus not on what the risk of the individual's needing care, but rather the consequences providing care to him or her would have on you and others providing it.

If this is done properly, he should understand that even though he believes he will not live a long life or even if he does, will not need care, the consequences to you and others could be severe. Please review the following talking points.

Talking points

Wife discussing the subject with her husband

"I am starting to think about the future and the possibility of my or your needing care as we get older."

> *"What do you mean?"*

"Have you thought about the consequences needing care over a period of years could have on our kids and the retirement portfolio?"

> *"Not really but we're not even 60 yet. Why worry now?"*

"I am starting to see the impact on my friends' lives when their parents need care."

> *"What if we don't live a long life or even if we do, don't get sick?"*

"That may happen, but my friends have told me that their parents didn't think they would live a long life or get sick even if they did. Look what happened to their children when they were wrong. I am concerned that if either of us needed care, it could have terrible consequences for our children."

> *"I don't want them to take care of us."*

"What choice will they have if we don't think about it? I am also worried that if you or I ever need care it would force us to reallocate income and assets to pay for it. The problem is that our portfolio is supposed to support our lifestyle. Think about what would happen if it had to be spent on care."

> *"I never thought about it like that."*

▼ N O T E S **Daughter discussing the subject with her father**

"Dad, I need to talk to you about the consequences living a long life and needing care will have on mom and us."

> *"I'm not going to live a long life — your grandfather died when he was 60 and I suspect the same will happen to me."*

"Dad, my guess is that your retirement portfolio is designed to pay out into your early nineties. That tells me you believe you could live a long life."

> *"It does, but that's to take care of your mother. I'm still not convinced that I will live that long."*

"That's my point: You may not live a long life, but if you do and need care over a period of years, the consequences to mom and the retirement plan could be devastating. You have to at least consider it."

> *"What if I never get sick?"*

"You may never need care, but if you did, it could place me in a difficult position."

> *"That's between your mother and me. Neither of us would want you to take care of us."*

"Honestly Dad, what choice would I have? Taking care of you will be very stressful for Mom. I can't stand by and see that happen. Think for a moment of any friends you have who have had the same issue when their Mom or Dad got sick."

> *"What do you think we should do?"*

A niece discussing the subject with her uncle

"Uncle Alan, I need to talk to you about the consequences living a long life and needing care will have on me and your other nieces and nephews."

> *"I'm not going to live a long life. My brother is already dead and there's a history of heart problems in the family."*

"Uncle Alan, my guess is that your retirement portfolio is designed to pay out into your early nineties. That tells me you believe you could live a long life."

> *"It does, but I still may be dead and even if I do live, I may never need care."*

"That's my point: You may not live a long life, but if you do and need care over a period of years, the consequences to all of us could be devastating"

> *"I wouldn't want you to take care of me. I can do it myself."*

"How? Have you considered that we won't have a choice?"

Types of Care: Everything You Need to Know

2

Levels of care 30

    Custodial care..30

        Activities of daily living (ADLs)...30

        Cognitive impairment...31

        Custodial care is most often given at home.................................31

    Skilled care..32

Types of care are determined by the extent of the illness.......................................32

    Home care 33

        Custodial care at home 33

        Skilled care at home 33

        Adult day care centers...33

    Assisted-living facilities..34

    Continuing Care Retirement Communities 35

    Institutional care..36

        Hospitals 36

        Nursing homes..36

▼ N O T E S   The previous chapter discussed the consequences of needing long-term care. This chapter will describe the types of care available and the places where it is provided.

How and where care is administered is the foundation of your long-term care plan. As you read about the different ways it can be delivered, think about the environment you or a family member would want. Most care discussed will be at home.

Levels of care

Long-term care, the assistance a sick or disabled person needs to go about the day, can be divided into two levels: *custodial care* (also known as *non-skilled care*) and *skilled care* (also referred to as *medical care*).

Custodial care

More than 90% of long-term care is custodial care. It is generally defined as assistance with activities of daily living (ADLs) or supervision needed by someone with a cognitive impairment.

Activities of daily living (ADLs)

Activities of daily living (ADLs) are the basic functions that as healthy, able adults, we often take for granted. For someone whose mobility is diminished by an illness or disability, ADLs are simple tasks that have become extremely difficult, or even impossible, without assistance. They include:

Bathing:	Getting in or out of a bathtub or shower and washing.
Eating:	Manipulating utensils and eating independently.

Dressing: Putting on clothes, being able to manipulate buttons and zippers.

Toileting: Using the toilet without assistance.

Continence: Maintaining bladder and bowel control.

Transferring: Moving from one place to another—from a bed to a chair, or from the kitchen table to the couch, for example.

Cognitive impairment

Cognitive impairment is generally defined as a deterioration or loss of intellectual capacity, including:

- short- or long-term memory;

- orientation as to person, place and time;

- deductive or abstract reasoning; and

- judgment as it relates to safety awareness.

Cognitive impairment does not necessarily lead to inability to perform ADLs. For example, an individual suffering from Alzheimer's disease may be able to perform ADLs until long into the course of his illness.

Custodial care is most often given at home

Whether care is needed because of diminished mobility or a cognitive impairment, most custodial care is provided outside of a medical setting, usually at home. *Formal care* is that administered by trained professionals, such as nurse's aides, professional personal caregivers and housekeepers. Assistance given by family members or close friends is referred to as *informal care*.

▼ N O T E S **Skilled care**

Skilled care is defined as care so inherently complex it can only be administered under a plan of care created by a doctor and executed by nurses or their equivalent.

Types of care are determined by the extent of the illness

When one thinks about long-term care services and facilities, it's best to view them on a continuum. In most cases, the effects of aging start slowly and gradually escalate. Think of someone in the early stages of Alzheimer's disease who is prone to misplacing things or forgetting names. As the disease progresses, he will experience increased confusion, encountering trouble doing daily tasks like grocery shopping and paying bills. Eventually, he will have difficulty dressing, eating and performing other ADLs.

The individual's initial care needs may be incidental and easily addressed at home by a spouse or family member. But as years pass and his health deteriorates, the level and type of care that is necessary becomes more complex. The individual patient may eventually require the help of professional aides and may someday need to be moved into a care facility.

As you read through the following descriptions of care services and facilities, consider all of them as you design your long-term care plan. Planning for all contingencies now will give you control over how and where care is delivered. Again, you may never need care, but if you do, your plan will allow you to maintain your independence while protecting the emotional and physical wellbeing of those you love.

Home care

Given a choice, most Americans will elect to age in place. That is, they will use whatever services become necessary to remain in their homes. Historically, aging in place was a practical alternative to nursing-home care, as long as the care needed was not too intensive and an informal caregiver (usually a family member) was available. But times have changed.

With the rise of dual-income households, yesterday's housewives, often relegated to caring for a parent or in-law, are today's earners. Many spend at least 40 hours a week at the workplace, making it difficult at best to provide care for mom or dad. Then there's the issue of geography. Families are spread apart today, and the once-common network of extended family living within an hour of one another is becoming rare.

Custodial care at home

The overwhelming amount of care in long-term care settings is *custodial* (*non-skilled*) in nature and is provided in a home setting. Caregivers are usually the spouses, assisted by children.

Skilled care at home

Because skilled care is more intensive, receiving this type of care at home usually requires house calls by medical professionals. Skilled home care may include a daily visit by a registered nurse who performs necessary medical procedures, or a weekly visit from a physical therapist to improve the patient's mobility.

Adult day care centers

People who suffer from light to moderate impairments and need supervision may benefit from adult day care centers

▼ NOTES (sometimes called *adult day centers*), a form of non-skilled care that is often provided in a community setting. Program participants can usually walk, but may need help with other activities of daily living.

Adult day centers serve as respite for the caregiver. For example, it allows the spouse of an Alzheimer's patient a few hours off, or it provides a way for an adult daughter to go to work during the day, knowing her impaired father is in a safe, stimulating environment.

Some adult day care centers share facilities with childcare centers because it is believed that children can stimulate people who suffer from dementia. In turn, the children learn valuable lessons from their elderly counterparts.

Assisted-living facilities

Assisted-living facilities supply varying levels of care for people who have some trouble with daily activities, but can, for the most part, still get through their daily routines. The care is provided in a secure, home-like environment where residents live in individual apartments. Meals and services are provided in central social rooms.

Because they're generally not subject to the same regulatory requirements as traditional nursing homes, assisted-living facilities can offer greater innovation in physical design, staffing arrangements and resident services. And since residents usually do not require skilled care, assisted-living facilities tend to employ well-trained, yet lower-cost paraprofessionals, although most of these facilities keep a nurse on call for residents who need limited health care.

Individual units, or apartments, within assisted-living facilities are typically rented, and cost varies, depending on geographic region. Costs are highest in the Northeast and on the West Coast, peaking in high-density cities like New York. Contact the Commission on Accreditation of Rehabilitation Facilities[1] or the Assisted Living Federation of America[2] for specific information about assisted living costs in your area.

Continuing Care Retirement Communities

A *continuing care retirement community (CCRC),* also known as a *life-care community,* is usually divided into three living components housed on one campus: an independent-living facility where there are no long-term care support services; an assisted-living facility; and a skilled nursing home. This built-in continuum of care allows seniors to age in a familiar setting with the comfort of knowing they have access to increasing levels of care as their needs develop.

While assisted-living residents pay rent, CCRC residents make a contract with the facility that outlines how they will pay for and receive care for the duration of their lives. CCRC residents pay an entrance or buy-in fee when they move in that typically ranges from $100,000 to $400,000, as well as monthly fees.

CCRCs have different policies regarding return of the entrance fee at residents' death or if they move. What the resident's estate receives back at his death depends on the facility. The standard in the industry is to return 90% of the original investment. Because of the costs and contracts involved, it is best to consult with an attorney or financial professional before considering this type of facility.

---

1 http://www.carf.org

2 http://www.alfa.org

▼ N O T E S **Institutional care**

Hospitals

Hospitals provide medical, not custodial care. They generally act as gateways to long-term care in another setting. If a patient is admitted to the hospital with a broken hip, he will be discharged after doctors determine that the fracture has been stabilized. If hospitalized for at least 72 hours, he qualifies for continued skilled or rehabilitative services for up to 100 days, paid for by Medicare.

Nursing homes

Nursing homes (also called *skilled nursing facilities*) provide round-the-clock medical care or rehabilitative services. The majority of nursing home admissions come from hospitals where the patient has been treated for a medical event. Further treatment or rehabilitation is conducted by the nursing home.

Despite their name, most of the long-term care that nursing homes provide is non-skilled care. In theory, the goal is to rehabilitate the patient so he can return home. However, many times nursing homes are the only option for individuals who require substantial assistance that cannot be provided in the community.

Nursing homes are licensed by both state and federal governments and must have qualified professionals on staff to attend to the needs of the patients.

The Best Long-Term Care Plan for You

3

Single, no children 39

Single with children 40

Married without children 42

Married with children 43

Second marriage with children 44

Divorced or widowed with children 46

Committed same-sex relationship 47

▼ N O T E S   At this point you should have a good idea of what long-term care is. You understand that the sick or disabled have many care options—from minimal, home-based assistance to full-service nursing home care, along with several variations in between. You also understand that when someone needs long-term care, it can negatively affect the emotional, physical and financial wellbeing of the entire family. The first question is: At what age should you start thinking about the subject?

As previously mentioned in Chapter 2, it makes sense to start the process when you are in your mid to late fifties. Here is a recap:

1. You tend to focus more intently on retirement and whether your portfolio will be sufficient to fund it.

2. You begin to see your friends or acquaintances get sick and realize that these things could actually happen to you.

3. You may be going through long-term care with your parents or in-laws, and now see what the impact of not having a plan is on caregivers and retirement portfolios.

You certainly can wait to put together a plan for care later on in life. The problem may be that if long-term care insurance is considered as a way to fund the plan, you may not qualify because of your health.

This chapter outlines your first step toward creating a long-term care plan. That plan has three goals:

1. Allow you to remain in the community for as long as possible.

2. Minimize the impact providing care to you will have on your family.

3. Preserve your retirement portfolio so it can continue to generate income to support your post-retirement lifestyle and keep your promises to you family and community.

The general plan may be the same for everyone, but different personal or family circumstances call for different approaches. What follows is a series of sample plans based on my more than twenty years of experience observing family dynamics. Obviously, every family is different, but the scenarios will give you a starting point for achieving the above goals. You may never need care in the future, but having a plan in place now will prove invaluable if care is needed.

Single, no children

Staying at home is very difficult for those who are single with no children, because there is no infrastructure—no spouse, children or grandchildren—to provide care. It may be possible to remain at home if the person needing care has siblings, nephews or nieces, or enough money to afford formal home care. You may not want your family members to provide your care, but what choice will they have if they see you starting to fail? That's why you may want to consider the following.

- **Assisted-living facility**

    An assisted-living facility may seem appropriate, but in my experience, few people want to move from their homes. The long-term care industry recognizes this, which is why marketing efforts promoting these facilities are focused on the adult children of those who need care, rather than the care recipients themselves. Even those who consider assisted living often put off the decision to move into the facility because they feel they can live independently a little longer. When the person needing care waits too long to make a decision, the result is often that the decision is taken out of his hands by a physician or someone appointed to make decisions for him.

- **Continuing care retirement community**

  This type of community setting makes the most sense for someone in this situation. Your plan then is to consider moving into the community while you are still healthy and enjoy full independence and autonomy. If you begin to require help with activities of daily living, trained staff is available to keep you safe and independent. If you need additional care, the assisted-living facility is available on the same campus. If your condition continues to worsen, the nursing home on campus is also available.

Single with children

For those who are single or widowed with children, remaining at home may be an option. However, the adult children will probably play a large role in keeping you there. This may include frequent visits to provide care, or more drastic steps, such as a child moving into your home, or moving in with a child and his or her family. If children live out of state, your ability to remain home is severely limited.

If what I just described seems like a viable option for your family, be sure to discuss potential care arrangements now. Determine who will carry the caregiving load and how out-of-

town siblings can help contribute to care. As a family, consider   N O T E S ▼
ways to lessen the care burden, such as:

- **Home-care services**

    Determine how home services might play a role in
    providing care. What's available in your community?
    What are the costs of formal care? These profession-
    als can work with the adult children to come up with a
    care plan that provides a high level of care to you while
    accommodating the children's schedules.

- **Assisted-living facility**

    This option makes sense if the illness progresses.
    Deciding when it's time to move into an assisted-living
    facility will be difficult for caregivers and you alike.
    Again, by planning ahead, you, as a family, can make
    decisions about when a parent needs to move into as-
    sisted living before a care need exists. Come up with
    moving triggers such as "when Mom needs round-the-
    clock supervision" or "when Dad can't take a bath by
    himself." These triggers are not written in stone, but
    discussing the issues before you're entangled in the
    emotional grip of caregiving can make the decision-
    making process less painful if care is needed.

- **Continuing care retirement community**

    This option makes the most sense for families who are
    unable or unwilling to provide care, or for parents who
    don't want their children involved in caregiving activi-
    ties.

Married without children

In this situation, a couple's first instinct might be that the sick spouse will be able to stay home far longer because the other spouse, who is not chronically ill, will be able to provide care. That may or may not be possible. The relatively healthy spouse will likely be in the same age bracket as the sick one, and possibly frail. If so, it will be next to impossible to provide the physical care (bathing, toileting, etc.) that will become necessary. What if someone falls?

- **Home-care services**

  Home care will be a lifesaver for couples who want to keep the sick spouse home. Before care is needed, it is essential to become familiar with home care services in your area. When care becomes necessary, don't hesitate to call these services early in an illness. The sooner the well spouse acknowledges that he or she cannot perform the constant work required, the less likely the well spouse will get hurt in the process, keeping everyone healthier and at home longer.

- **Adult day care services**

  Especially in cases of cognitive impairment, a sick spouse's ability to remain home will be greatly enhanced when home care is combined with adult day services.

- **Assisted-living facility**

  This type of facility makes sense as the illness gets the better of both the sick spouse and the spouse providing care. If you're the well spouse, listen to caregivers if they suggest it may be time to consider this option, even if you don't think it's the right move. What makes the decision easier is that all facilities allow the well spouse to move in.

- **Continuing care retirement community**

  Again, moving into an apartment on a CCRC campus while one is still healthy is often an ideal choice for everyone involved. If needed, care is available. If not, a couple can enjoy living in a lively, independent community.

Married with children

Those who are married with children have the best odds of staying home longer because, in theory, there is a built-in infrastructure of children who can share the responsibility of providing care with the well spouse. The operative phrase, of course, is "in theory."

While this infrastructure may exist, having children provide care may be unrealistic. What if the children live far away or have growing families? What impact will a child's providing care have on his or her relationship with siblings who do not? Think about the position in which the children will be placed financially if they need to help pay for your care.

- **Home-care services**

  Investigate home care services, especially as you advance into your sixties and seventies. Start a dialogue between doctors, family and service providers to determine what role they can play in your care. How much time can the adult children contribute? How much care can the well spouse handle? Where can the service provider fill the gaps?

- **Assisted-living facility**

  This type of care makes sense if your illness progresses. If your spouse is sick, listen to his caregivers if they suggest it may be time to consider this option, even if you don't think it's the right move.

- **Continuing care retirement community**

  This long-term care option makes the most sense for those who are married with children, because it doesn't require the adult children to restructure their lives to take care of their parents. The parents can remain on campus, regardless of their care needs, and a well spouse won't shoulder the entire burdened of caring for a sick spouse.

Second marriage with children

Of all the families with which I have worked, perhaps the most sensitive situations involved second marriages, particularly those where one or both spouses have children from previous marriages. If this describes your situation, here are some issues that should be discussed:

1. What role will the adult children of the ill spouse play in providing care? You need to state your intentions clearly as to who will provide it and on which authority. Make sure you have a *health care proxy* and that your children are aware of it; this document will govern how and what care you will receive if you become unable to make these decisions yourself.

2. How do you plan on paying for care at home, in assisted living, etc? Is there a discrepancy in income and assets? If so, it may turn out that your funds may have

to be used to pay for your spouse's care or vice-versa. That will almost immediately get the attention of the contributing spouse's children.

3. If the patient's spouse is paying for his care, how will the care be funded if the paying spouse dies prior to the sick spouse? I strongly recommend that a couple in a second marriage draft durable powers of attorney that indicate who will make these and other decisions if the spouses can no longer do so themselves.

- **Home-care services**

  Staying home is a viable option, but you have to discuss which of the children will provide care. It may be a better idea not to have any of them involved, because of the potentially delicate relationship with your spouse.

- **Assisted-living facility**

  An assisted-living facility makes sense if a spouse's illness progresses after he receives care at home. I recommend that when the decision to enter an assisted-living facility is made, the well spouse consult with the ill spouse's children. This is particularly important if the well spouse doesn't have much of a relationship with them. Excluding them puts the well spouse's authority at risk. Ideally, this situation will be discussed among all parties — both spouses and all the children — long before either parent requires assisted living.

- **Continuing care retirement community**

  Because it requires a large upfront investment, a continuing care retirement community may raise issues with some of the children. Questions to discuss include:

1. Whose money is being used?

2. Has the couple made arrangements to support a surviving spouse if the deceased spouse was paying for the CCRC?

3. Does the CCRC return money at death? If so, who will receive this money?

For couples in second marriages, purchasing a long-term care insurance policy is critical to the success of your plan. A comprehensive discussion of such insurance is the subject of Chapter 6.

Divorced or widowed with children

If you are divorced and have a working relationship with your former spouse, I strongly suggest you sit down with him or her to discuss long-term care issues. Here is a discussion a close friend had with his former spouse.

"Ellen, do you think you could live a long life?"

"I hope to."

"It's possible that you may need care in the future — fair statement?"

"Maybe — it's not unreasonable."

"I assume that if you do need care, you would want to stay at home?"

"Absolutely."

"That's going to be very difficult unless one or more of the kids moves in with you."

"That's not fair to any of them. I don't want that. What do you think I should do?"

After discussing the options in this section, they decided that a continuing care retirement community would make the most sense for her as she aged. Once she decided *where* and *how* she would receive care, they figured out how to fund her plan, which will be discussed in Chapter 4.

Committed same-sex relationship

Couples in same sex relationships have to consider the availability of support from their families. They may or may not have adequate infrastructure to support care over a period of time. Here are some considerations:

- Who will make medical decisions for each of the people in the relationship? Neither partner should assume it is the other one. This must be discussed while the couple is healthy; otherwise it opens the door for relatives or children to impose their ideas of where and how care should be given. Both partners need a health care proxy—today.

- Who will make financial decisions for each of the people in the relationship? Again, neither partner should assume it is the other. Failure to draft a durable power of attorney is a prescription for a legal battle to control funds and ultimately care.

Next, let's address the question of where care would be provided.

- ### Home-care services

  Staying home may be difficult if the healthy partner needs to work and there is limited support from family. However, it is possible if the plan includes creating an infrastructure consisting of professional home-care workers and homemakers supported by adult day care.

- ### Assisted-living facility

  An assisted-living facility makes sense if either partner's illness progresses. It is strongly recommended that the sick partner consult with his relatives and children, if he has any. This is particularly important if you don't have much of a relationship with each other's families. Cutting them out of the loop puts you on the fast track to a legal challenge of your authority.

  Here are some other issues that must be discussed if you choose an assisted-living facility:

  - Whose money is being used to pay the monthly fee?

  - What arrangements are there to continue paying for care if the healthy partner, who is paying for it, predeceases the sick partner?

- ### Continuing care retirement community

  Continuing care retirement community may create issues with the relatives or children, because it requires a large upfront investment. Here are some issues to be addressed:

  - Whose money is being used?

48

- What arrangements are there to continue paying for care if the healthy partner, who is paying for it, predeceases the sick partner?

- Does the CCRC facility return money at death? If yes, who will receives it, the surviving partner or the relatives?

Whatever decisions you make, make them sooner rather than later. Doing so assures that you will be taken care of in the least restrictive environment while minimizing the impact providing care will have on your family and finances.

The above plans are meant to offer a framework. It is strongly recommended that you consult with a long-term care professional who can help you craft the right plan for your circumstances. Refer to Chapter 8 for more information on finding a qualified long-term care specialist.

Next, we will explore the best options to finance your plan.

Funding Your Plan 4

Paying for your plan 52
Self-funding.. 52
    Modest wealth: assets under $800,000 54
    Very comfortable: assets of $800,000–$2,000,000 55
    Wealthy: Assets in excess of $2,000,000 57
        Life insurance..58
        Home equity 59
Medicare 61
    Medicare *vs* Medicaid.. 61
    Medicare basics 61
    Medicare Part A 62
        Inpatient hospitalization 63
        Skilled nursing-home care 63
        Home care services 64
        Coverage.. 64
        "But my friend said Medicare paid for her Mom's home care"..................... 66
    Medicare Part B 67
        Will Part B pay for custodial care at home?.............................68
    Medicare Part C: Medicare Advantage 68
    Medicare Part D: The Prescription Drug Benefit 68
Veterans' benefits 69
    Veterans Health Administration and long-term care 70
    Eligibility..70
    Will the VA pay for custodial care? 73
    Benefits for long-term care based on financial eligibility 74
    Funding is limited 75
    The bottom line for veterans 75

▼ N O T E S **Paying for your plan**

Once you have established a long-term care plan, the logical next step is to determine how it will be paid for. Please keep in mind that the care is custodial (non-skilled) in nature. That means assistance with your activities of daily living or supervision necessitated by a cognitive impairment.

Long-term care services are expensive. Here's a brief survey of what it costs to keep you or a loved one safe in 2007, according to Genworth Financial, an insurance company which surveys long-term care costs each year:[1]

- The average annual national cost of private room in a nursing home is $74,806 ($205 a day).

- The average monthly cost of a one-bedroom unit in an assisted living facility is $2,714 ($89 per day).

- The average hourly rate for a certified home health aide is $32.37, and for an unlicensed health aide—$18.57.

Your default plan will likely be to remain independent in the community. This chapter investigates what will pay to support your efforts at home, or if you need them, assisted living or skilled nursing home care.

Self-funding

The problem with self-funding is that it doesn't come from your life savings, it comes from a retirement portfolio. There is a significant difference between the two.

---

1 Genworth Financial, Inc., Richmond, VA:
Genworth Financial 2007 Cost of Care Survey
http://longtermcare.genworth.com/overview/cost_of_care.jsp

Most people believe that life savings can be used for any number of things. If told that they may have to pay for care from life savings they might ask, "Do you think there is enough?" If told, however, that the only way their care may be paid for is with funds from their retirement portfolio, the answer is more likely to be "I am counting on that to fund my retirement."

People with resources live a lifestyle at retirement, and that lifestyle is not one of subsistence. If they have a portfolio of $2 million, the income is likely accounted for to support their passions such as golf, sailing and traveling. It is also being used to keep continuing commitments to their family and community. It is not likely there is a lot left over. Make a quick note of your estimated income and expenses at retirement in this table:

Income	Expenses

You may believe that you have the resources to pay for your care over a period of years. That may or may not be the case. Let's look at three situations based on net worth:

Modest: assets under $800,000

Very comfortable: assets of $800,000–$2,000,000

Wealthy: assets over $2,000,000

▼ NOTES **Modest wealth: assets under $800,000**

You could possibly pay for care over a period of years from you retirement portfolio. Rather than focus on assets, however, I would like you to think about income. Your lifestyle and ability to keep financial commitments to your family and community during retirement will likely be paid for from income generated from your Social Security retirement benefits, pension (if any), and the payout of qualified funds such as IRAs, 401(k) or 403(b).

May I suggest that you use the table above to calculate what your estimated income and expenses will be at retirement. My experience tells me there will be very little, if anything, income left after the expenses. Here's what I tell my clients:

"I think you understand that your retirement portfolio will generate income to support the things you want to do after you retire. Here's the problem: I don't believe that, should you need care, the income will be sufficient to support both care and your lifestyle at the same time. That likely means you will have to substantially cut back on your financial commitments. I'm not sure that's what you want."

For the first time, clients begin to understand that, although they believe they may never become frail or sick and need care, the consequences to their lifestyle if they do could be catastrophic.

Conclusion

If you or your parents have a modest net worth and need care over a period of time, it is likely that income, otherwise allocated to support your lifestyle and keep promises to family and community, will have to be reallocated to pay for it. If the illness continues long enough, there is the very real possibility that principal may have to be invaded, threatening the financial viability of a surviving spouse and others who may depend on that income.

Very comfortable: assets of $800,000–$2,000,000

Here are some beliefs my wealthier clients share regarding self-funding the cost of care. Each comes with its own inherent problems:

- Mindset: *"I have about $1.5 million dollars. My advisor told me that's more than enough to pay for care."*

  The problem: There's little doubt that a family can pay for care out-of-pocket with that size portfolio. But if this is how you plan to fund care, consider the following:

  - You likely have a considerable amount of assets in a tax-deferred IRA, 401(k) or 403(b) funds. Paying for care from these assets will trigger a federal tax as high as 35% plus whatever your state tax is.

  - If you have to pay for your care by selling assets with a low cost basis (the value of the asset when you bought it), the sale will trigger a tax on the capital gain (sale price less cost basis).

  - As stated earlier, lifestyle is likely supported by your income stream. Diverting it to pay for care may have a serious impact on your family's retirement lifestyle.

  Let's assume your portfolio has declined in a down market. It's likely that, like most, you will resist the normal instinct to liquidate because you correctly believe the market will recover. If you don't sell, in effect you will sustain only a paper loss.

My experience has shown that if a person needs care, assets are likely to be liquidated in a down market—not because the family needs the funds right away, but rather they are concerned the market may continue to decline when those assets are needed. A paper loss is now turned into a real loss of principal.

- Mindset: *"If I get sick, I won't be able to do the things I want to do in retirement anyway, so the money I save can be used to pay for care."*

The problem: It's not just your lifestyle, it's your family's as well.

I met a woman whose family was well off financially. They belonged to an exclusive country club, summered in Maine, and loved to travel. Her mother was diagnosed with Alzheimer's. At some point she asked for my assistance about qualifying for Medicaid.

As I have explained in this book, I told her that transferring assets would create a substantial tax liability. I also told her that, given the estate, the family would never run out of funds.

It didn't matter.

She told me that she had no idea how long her mother would need care and how much it was going to cost. They were very concerned there may not be enough to pay for care and support her mother's lifestyle, which meant spending time at the club with children and grandchildren, continuing to keep their house in Maine and helping grandchildren with education costs.

Telling them there was enough did not assuage their fears.

Her mother lived for eight years. It turned out that the family was still left with substantial assets. I asked them whether their advisor had recommended long-term care insurance. "We talked about it but the advisor told my parents they had enough," I was told. Are you upset at the advisor, I inquired. "Yes," they replied, "about two things. First, we had no plan in place and didn't understand the stress of providing care. Second, even though we knew intellectually there was enough, it didn't matter when we started to spend the money."

Postscript to the story: The children purchased long-term care insurance for themselves.

Conclusion

Clearly you can self-insure the risk. But in my experience self-insuring means that the individual doesn't believe the event will happen. I suggest instead you look at consequences. Consider the story above; talk to those who have had an experience with long-term care, and they will tell that there is no such thing as enough when you start paying out-of-pocket.

Wealthy: Assets in excess of $2,000,000

Income allocation and liquidity arguments are ineffective when discussing paying for care. If you have a substantial net worth, go ahead and self-insure. But make sure to carefully consider the consequences of your decision.

I have seen families with far more than $2,000,000 decide not to self-insure and instead purchase long-term care insurance. Here's what I found out:

- Almost all had a prior experience with long-term care.

- Wealthy people do not assess risk; they assess consequences.

- They still deeply believe the risk of their needing care is very low (remember, reasonable people do not live their lives in fear). However, they now see how the consequences to their family and finances are likely to be catastrophic without a plan of care and insurance to protect it.

Other assets that can be used to pay for care:

Life insurance

Most people associate life insurance with death, not long-term care, but some life insurance policies can be an important source of personal funds. Permanent life insurance in any form (whole life, universal life and variable life) creates a cash value that may be used to pay for long-term care costs (in the form of accelerated benefits). Many policies today also include a living-benefit provision that authorizes the payment of the policy's face amount, or a portion of it, in the event of the policyholder's permanent confinement in a long-term care facility.

Some insurance carriers offer policyholders the right to accelerate benefits. Generally, companies:

- allow only a portion of the death benefit to be drawn on, and may apply interest.

- pay less than 50% of the death benefit.

- still lapse policies whose holders do not continue to pay premiums.

Some life insurance policies that are no longer needed may be sold for more money than you'd receive by surrendering the policy to the insurance company. This transaction, in which the assignment of a life insurance owner's death benefit is exchanged for a lump sum payout now, is called a *life settlement*. There are some general guidelines for life settlements:

- The policyholder has a life expectancy of 12 years or less;

- is over age 55; and

- owns a policy with a cash surrender value and a face value above a certain minimum, usually at least $100,000.

The cash generated from a life settlement could be used to pay for long-term care services. The question is, do you really want to cash in your policy to pay for care?

The above are general guidelines. Please check your individual life insurance policy for terms and conditions.

Home equity

The equity in a home can be substantial, especially if the house was purchased many years earlier and the mortgage is paid off. This can be a valuable source of funds to cover long-term care costs. There are two ways to tap into this money:

- **Home equity loans:** Significant drawbacks limit their appeal. Will the borrower have future income to pay the loan back? What if a spouse whose income was intended to be used for the repayment dies prematurely?

- **Home equity conversion mortgages (HECMs or reverse mortgages)**: This program allows homeowners to tap into the equity in their home without the need to pay it back during their lifetime. Whatever is borrowed accrues interest to be paid back along with the principal at either death or the sale of the home.

The program could be useful in generating income to pay for long-term insurance, or, if you don't qualify for such insurance, pay for care in the community, should you need it.

Home equity conversion mortgages can be used by homeowners who are 62 years old or older. Borrowers may choose one of five payment options:

1. Monthly income for life.

2. Monthly income for a fixed period of time.

3. A line of credit.

4. A combination of lifetime income and a line of credit.

5. A combination of income for a fixed period of time with a line of credit.

The borrower remains the owner of the home and may sell it and move at any time, keeping the sales proceeds that exceed the mortgage balance. He cannot be forced to sell the home to pay off the mortgage, even if the mortgage balance grows to exceed the value of the property.

If the loan exceeds the value of the property when it is paid, the borrower (or the heirs) will owe no more than the value of the property. Federal Housing Administration (FHA) insurance will cover any balance due the lender.

As part of the HECM program, the federal Department of Housing and Urban Development (HUD) provides free reverse-mortgage counseling for persons considering using such an instrument. The toll-free information phone line is 1-888-466-3487.

Medicare

Medicare *vs* Medicaid

Federal law established both Medicare and Medicaid in 1965. Because the names are so alike, it's easy to confuse these two government health care programs. However, there are distinct differences:

- **Medicare** is a federal health insurance program financed exclusively by recipients through payroll taxes. Your state does not contribute to the program. It is called an entitlement program because you are entitled to benefits, regardless of assets and income, by paying into the program during your working years.

- **Medicaid** is also a health insurance program, but it is reserved for those who are financially needy. It is a joint partnership between your state and the federal government.

Medicare basics

The Medicare program, administered by the Centers for Medicare and Medicaid Services (CMS), consists of four parts:

- **Parts A & Part B, Original Medicare:** This basic plan requires the beneficiary to contribute to cost of care in the form of deductibles and co-insurance. These obligations can be covered by a Medicare supplement;

- **Part C, Medicare Advantage:** Medicare Advantage plans are offered by private health insurance carriers instead of Part A and Part B. They usually offer additional benefits (generally, for an additional premium) and lower copayments. Part C subscribers have to continue paying their Part B premiums. Medicare Advantage plans can be based on HMO (Health Maintenance Organization), PPO (Preferred Provider Organization), or fee-for-service models.

- **Part D:** Medicare Prescription Drug Plan.

Regardless of the plan, as you will see, Medicare covers little custodial care. Here are Medicare's own words:

> *"Medicare also doesn't pay for help with activities of daily living or other care that most people can do themselves. Some examples of activities of daily living include eating, bathing, dressing, and using the bathroom. Medicare will help pay for skilled nursing or home health care if you meet certain conditions."* [2]

Medicare Part A

What's covered:

- Inpatient hospital care

- Skilled nursing-home care (limited to stays of up to 100 days)

- Skilled home health care

- Hospice care

- Blood transfusions

---

2 http://www.medicare.gov/LongTermCare/Static/Medicare.asp

Inpatient hospitalization

Medicare Part A covers reasonable charges for semiprivate rooms in accredited hospitals. It covers only charges billed by the hospital; it does not cover physician, surgeon or anesthesiologist services (those are covered through Medicare Part B.)

Benefit limits are applied to each benefit period. A new benefit period begins after the patient has been out of the hospital for at least 60 days. Full hospital charges are covered for the first 60 days after the patient has met a deductible.

After 60 days in the hospital, Part A coverage scales down. After the 90th day of hospitalization, the coverage stops. However, Medicare beneficiaries have an additional 60-day lifetime reserve that they may use.

Hospitals generally provide complex medical care. Their job is to stabilize the medical condition that caused the admission. Once that has been accomplished, the patient is discharged, either home or to a skilled nursing home for further treatment.

Hospitals operate under the so-called Prospective Payment System (PPS). Medicare Part A pays a predetermined rate (similar to a flat fee) for inpatient hospital care based on set criteria (referred to as *diagnostic-related groupings* or *DRGs*). If the facility can stabilize the patient for less than what it received from Medicare, it keeps the difference. If it spends more than Medicare pays, the hospital must absorb the excess. This system all but eliminates the possibility that a Medicare patient will receive anything other than skilled care.

Skilled nursing-home care

The benefits provided through Part A cover up to 100 days of post-hospitalization skilled nursing care for patients hospital-

▼ N O T E S

ized for more than 72 hours and who are moved to the facility within 30 days. They pay only for medical or rehabilitative care. Generally, patients stay in the skilled nursing facility for fewer than 30 days on Medicare's skilled-care coverage.

Home care services

Part A does cover home-care services, but only under limited conditions. Here is how you qualify:

1. Your doctor must decide that you need medical (skilled) care at home, and make a plan for your care at home.

2. You must need at least one of the following: intermittent skilled nursing care, physical therapy, speech-language therapy, or occupational therapy.

3. The home health agency caring for you must be approved by the Medicare program.

4. You must be *homebound*—able to leave home only with considerable and taxing effort—or normally unable to leave home unassisted at all. A Medicare home care recipient may leave home for medical treatment or short, infrequent absences for non-medical reasons, such as a trip to the barber or to attend a religious service. Use of adult day care doesn't prevent you from receiving home health care under Medicare.

Coverage

If you qualify for Medicare Part A, it will cover:

• Skilled nursing care on a part-time or intermittent basis. Skilled nursing care includes services and care that can be performed safely and correctly only by a licensed nurse (either a registered nurse or a licensed practical nurse).

- Home health aide services on a part-time or intermittent basis. A home health aide doesn't have a nursing license. The aide provides services that give additional support to the nurse. These services include help with personal care such as bathing, using the bathroom, or dressing. These types of services don't require the skills of a licensed nurse. However, Medicare doesn't cover home health aides who provide custodial care unless you are also receiving skilled care or other therapy.

- Physical therapy, including exercise to regain movement and strength in a body area, and training on how to use special equipment or do daily activities, like how to get in and out of a wheelchair or bathtub.

- Speech-language therapy (pathology services), including exercise to regain and strengthen speech skills.

- Occupational therapy to help you become able to do usual daily activities by yourself. You may continue to receive occupational therapy even if you no longer need other skilled care, if it is ordered by your doctor.

- Medical social services to help you with social and emotional concerns related to your illness. This might include counseling or help in finding resources in your community.

- Certain medical supplies like wound dressings, but not prescription drugs or biologicals.

- Durable medical equipment such as a wheelchair or walker.

- FDA (Food and Drug Administration)-approved inject-able osteoporosis drugs in certain circumstances.

However, Medicare will not pay for care that is long-term. Medicare pays providers a predetermined amount, similarly to how hospitals are reimbursed. Medicare will pay a home health care provider a set amount based on the patient's diagnosis, and not on the amount of time spent or services provided. In short, there is no incentive to provide more services.

Medicare will not cover the following services:

- Round-the-clock care at home.

- Meals delivered to your home.

- Homemaker services like shopping, cleaning, and laundry.

- Personal care given by home health aides like bathing, dressing, and using the bathroom, when this is the only care you need.

"But my friend said Medicare paid for her Mom's home care"

One reason people think Medicare provides custodial care is because in the past it likely did. Home health care agencies realized that many potential clients couldn't afford home care unless Medicare paid for it. They took advantage of vague regulations defining skilled and rehabilitative services to give patients the benefit of the doubt. Often this resulted in extensive services for custodial care. There was also a financial incentive: providers were paid on a fee-for-service basis. The more care they provided, the more money they received.

This changed after the passage of the Balanced Budget Act of 1997. As of 1998, home health care providers are paid on a flat-fee basis and home care visits are generally capped at 100

days. Providers are carefully watched by Medicare and are subject to substantial penalties if they try to bill for custodial care.

Medicare Part B

Medicare Part B is a voluntary program that supplements Part A coverage. Medicare beneficiaries may elect Part B when they become eligible for Part A. Part B requires a monthly premium ($93.50 in 2007) that increases based on your income. Medicare Part B premiums are deducted from the beneficiary's monthly Social Security retirement check.

In many ways, Medicare Part B resembles major medical insurance. It shifts the costs of incidental medical care to the policyholder through deductibles and coinsurance, and cosmetic and nonessential elective surgeries usually are not covered.

Benefits offered under Part B that are subject to deductible and coinsurance limits include:

- Physician services

- Outpatient hospital care

- Surgical services and supplies

- Physical and speech therapy

- Ambulance trips

- Diagnostic tests

- Durable medical equipment (including wheelchairs, walkers and hospital beds)

- Prosthetic devices

- Blood Transfusions

▼ N O T E S   **Will Part B pay for custodial care at home?**

Medicare Part B covers the same services as Part A (see above).

Medicare Part C: Medicare Advantage

The Balanced Budget Act of 1997 included changes to the Medicare program. The new law included a section called Medicare + Choice that provided new health plan options. Under the Medicare Modernization Act of 2003, Medicare + Choice was given a new name: Medicare Advantage.

Medicare Advantage provides beneficiaries alternatives to Parts A and B, including Medicare Managed Care Plans, Medicare HMOs, Medicare PPOs, Medicare Special Needs Plans and Medicare Private Fee-for-Service Plans.

Most of these plans tout additional benefits and lower copayments, compared to traditional Medicare Parts A and B.

What's important to understand is that, like Medicare Parts A and B, Medicare Advantage is limited to skilled (acute) medical care. This is simply a program that provides beneficiaries with cost savings or additional options in selecting their physicians. It doesn't pay for long-term care services other than the skilled home-care services described on page 64.

Medicare Part D: The Prescription Drug Benefit

Starting on January 1, 2006, Medicare beneficiaries, regardless of income, health status, or their use of prescription drugs, became entitled to prescription drug coverage. Medicare contracts with private companies to offer a variety of coverage options; the more benefits, the higher the cost. The participant picks a plan that best meets his current prescription needs. Although this plan is voluntary, a penalty applies per

each month the beneficiary delays enrolling, in the amount of
1% of the national average plan cost for that month.

Here is a summary of how the plan works:

- An enrollee pays a monthly premium (which varies depending on the plan chosen, but is around $35) in addition to any premium for Medicare Part B.

- Regardless of which plan the enrollee chooses, he pays the first $250 per year for prescriptions (some plans may cover this deductible).

- The participant pays 25% of yearly drug costs from $250 to $2,250 (up to $500) and the plan pays the other 75% (up to $1,500).

- The participant pays 100% of drug costs from $2,250 to $5,100, or until total out-of-pocket costs reach $3,600 ($250 deductible + $500 out-of-pocket + $2,850 during the gap, known as the "donut hole").

- The participant then pays only 5% of drug costs for the rest of the calendar year after having spent a total of $3,600 out-of-pocket, and the insurer then pays the rest. This is known as the the "catastrophic benefit."

Enrollees with limited income and assets who are, however, not eligible for Medicaid, may qualify for additional assistance that would pay for around 95% of drug costs.

Veterans' benefits

Many of my clients believed that the U.S. Department of Veterans' Affairs (the VA) would pay for their veteran parent's care, but that didn't happen.

▼ NOTES   The VA is comprised of three organizations: the Veterans' Health Administration, the Veterans' Benefits Administration, and the National Cemetery Administration. The first two provide limited assistance to veterans needing long-term care, albeit in different forms.

Veterans Health Administration and long-term care

The VHA is an organization that, for the most part, provides health care to eligible veterans. Limited custodial (non-skilled) benefits are available, but they're generally rationed because of inadequate funding. Here's a basic description of how the VHA program works:

Eligibility

Any veteran who was honorably discharged from military service is eligible for the VA Medical Benefits package. Veterans who served after Sept. 8, 1980 must have performed two years of active duty.

VA funding for health care is limited. As a result, the VA can provide services only to a limited number of enrollees. To determine who can access benefits first, the VA prioritizes veterans based on the extent of their service-related injuries. In other words, the VA gives preferential treatment to those with the most severe service-related issues, not those with the most critical general health problems. Once veterans are enrolled, they generally receive the same services. Here's a breakdown of the priority groups:[3]

- Priority Group 1: Veterans with service-connected disabilities rated 50% or more disabling, or veterans

---

3   U.S. Department of Veterans Affairs
    http://www.va.gov/healtheligibility/eligibility/PriorityGroups.asp

determined by the VA to be unemployable due to
service-connected conditions.

- Priority Group 2: Veterans with service-connected disabilities rated 30% or 40% disabling.

- Priority Group 3: Veterans with service-connected disabilities rated 10% or 20% disabling, veterans who are former POWs, veterans awarded the Purple Heart, veterans whose discharge was for a disability that began in the line of duty, veterans who are disabled because of VA treatment or participation in a VA vocational rehabilitation program.

- Priority Group 4: Veterans who are receiving aid and attendance or housebound benefits (on pension) from the VA, veterans who have been determined by the VA to be catastrophically disabled.

- Priority Group 5: Veterans receiving VA pension benefits, veterans who are eligible for Medicaid programs, veterans with income and assets below VA Means Test Thresholds.

- Priority Group 6: Veterans with 0% service-connected conditions, but receiving VA compensation, veterans seeking care only for disorders relating to Ionizing Radiation and Project 112/SHAD, veterans seeking care for Agent Orange Exposure during service in Vietnam, veterans seeking care for Gulf War Illness or for conditions related to exposure to environmental contaminants during service in the Persian Gulf, veterans of World War I or the Mexican Border War, veterans who served in combat in a war after the Gulf War or during a period of hostility after November 11, 1998 for two years following discharge or release from the military.

- Priority Group 7: Veterans who agree to pay a specified copay with income and/or net worth above the VA Income Threshold and income below the Geographic Means Test Threshold.

    - Subpriority A: Noncompensable 0% service-connected veterans who were enrolled in the VA Health Care System on a specified date and who have remained enrolled since that date.

    - Subpriority C: Non-service-connected veterans who were enrolled in the VA Health Care System on a specified date and who have remained enrolled since that date.

    - Subpriority E: Noncompensable 0% service-connected veterans not included in Subpriority a above. The VA is not currently using Subpriority E.

    - Subpriority G: Non-service-connected veterans not included in Subpriority C above. The VA is not currently using Subpriority G.

- Priority Group 8: Veterans who agree to pay specified copay with income and/or net worth above the VA Means Test Threshold and the Geographic Means Test Threshold.

    - Subpriority A: Noncompensable 0% service-connected veterans enrolled as of January 16, 2003 and who have remained enrolled since that date.

    - Subpriority C: Non-service-connected veterans enrolled as of January 16, 2003 and who have remained enrolled since that date.

- Subpriority E: Noncompensable 0% service-connected veterans applying for enrollment after January 16, 2003.

- Subpriority G: Non-service-connected veterans applying for enrollment after January 16, 2003. Effective January 17, 2003, the VA suspended *new* enrollment of veterans assigned to Priority Group 8 (the VA's lowest priority group, consisting of higher-income veterans). If you are a veteran enrolling for the first time on or after January 17, 2003, and your income exceeds the current year income threshold, you are not eligible for enrollment at this time. Veterans enrolled in Priority Group 8 on or before January 16, 2003, will remain enrolled and continue to be eligible for the full-range of VA health care benefits.[4]

Will the VA pay for custodial care?

Veterans enrolled in the VA health care system are eligible for limited Home and Community Based Services (HCBS). These services may include hospice, adult day care, home health aides, homemaker services, and home-based primary care (HBPC) for persons with chronic disabling disease. However, copayment may be required.

The VHA provides nursing home services through three national programs:

- Nursing facilities owned and operated by the VA itself typically admit those with a 70% service-connected disability, those who require care due to a service con-

---

4 U.S. Department of Veterans Affairs
   http://www.va.gov/healtheligibility/Library/pubs/VAIncomeThresholds/

nected disability, or those requiring short-term reha-bilitative care. VA homes are not necessarily free of charge; they may require a copayment.

- State veterans' homes are a cooperative venture be-tween the VA and states where the VA provides funds to help build the home and pays a portion of the cost for veterans eligible for VA health care. The states, however, set eligibility criteria for admission. Typically, one-third of the cost of care is borne by the patient.

- The VA contract nursing home program is designed to meet the long-term care needs of veterans who may not be eligible or qualify for placement in a VA or state veterans home or if there is no VA or state home avail-able. Copayment may be required.

Benefits for long-term care based on financial eligibility

In 2007, the Veterans Benefits Administration may pay a separate Aid and Attendance benefit up to $1,470 a month to a qualifying veteran, $945 per month to a surviving spouse, or $1,743 per month to a couple to defray the expense of long-term care. To qualify, a wartime veteran (as defined by the VA), or the surviving spouse of a wartime veteran, must require assistance with ADLs, and meet an income threshold of $18,234 for a veteran without dependents. The threshold is $21,615 if a veteran has one dependent, and increases by $1,866 for each additional dependent. The threshold for a surviving spouse is $11,715, which increases to $13,976 with one dependent, and increases by $1,866 for each additional depen-dent.[5]

---

5 U.S. Department of Veterans Affairs
   http://www1.va.gov/opa/pressrel/pressrelease.cfm?id=1265

Funding is limited

A 2003 report from the U.S. General Accounting Office, "VA Long-Term Care: Service Gaps and Facility Restrictions Limit Veterans' Access to Non-Institutional Care," found that out of 139 VA facilities, 126 offered limited or no long-term care services, and what was offered was based on available funding.

Here are some other noteworthy facts:

- Of the $23 billion the VA spent on health care in fiscal year 2003, only $3.3 billion was allocated for long-term care services.

- A 1996 General Accounting Office report estimated that the VA paid for services for only 34,000 of the 235,000 veterans who needed care.

The bottom line for veterans

Ultimately, payment for custodial care is limited to people with severe service-connected disabilities and wartime veterans with limited income and assets. It is each veteran's responsibility to plan how to pay for his or her own care.

In 2001, the federal government, through the Office of Personnel Management, contracted with John Hancock and MetLife to provide long-term care insurance to federal employees and their families.[6] The creation of long-term care insurance for military personnel (among others) underscores the reality that the VA is primarily a health care provider. For more on the program go to Chapter 6.

---

6 http://www.opm.gov/insure/ltc

Medicaid

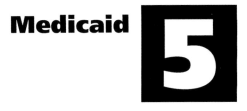

What is Medicaid 79

Medicaid *vs* Medicare 79

Covered services 80

    General medical services 80

    Long-term care services 80

Medicaid and home health care 81

Qualifying for Medicaid 82

    Medical eligibility 82

    Financial eligibility 82

        Assets 83

            The look-back period 85

            How a couple's assets are treated 86

            Community spouse resource allowance (CSRA) 86

            Prenuptial agreements 87

        Income 88

            How an individual's income is treated 88

            Cap states 88

            Miller trusts 89

            How a couple's income is treated 90

            Minimum monthly maintenance needs allowance (MMMNA) 90

        The Deficit Reduction Act of 2005 (DRA '05) 92

Planning for long-term care *vs* Medicaid planning 94

    Life estates 99

    Trusts 99

        Revocable trusts 100

        Irrevocable trusts 100

    "Medicaid-friendly" annuities 101

    Estate recovery 101

Illegal gifts 102

Still want to apply for Medicaid? 103

Medicaid planning in a crisis..103

Protecting a small business 104

If you have a disabled child: the supplemental-needs trust (SNT) 104

Protecting a primary residence...104

Choosing a lawyer 105

Interviewing a lawyer...106

What is Medicaid

Many people believe that Medicaid will pay for their care in the community or in facilities, if needed. That may not be the case.

Medicaid is a health care program available to those with limited income and assets. It is a joint venture between states and the federal government. In short, Medicaid is welfare. It's a safety net for millions of Americans who, for whatever reason, are not able to pay for their health care costs. To qualify, an applicant must meet eligibility standards.

The primary purpose of the program is to provide health care coverage for participants. It will, however, pay for custodial care in a skilled nursing home and limited services in the community, as this chapter will discuss. Also covered is how the program can be used in a crisis and what impact recent legislation signed into law by President George W. Bush on February 8, 2006 will have on eligibility.

Medicaid *vs* Medicare

Medicare is a federal health insurance program financed exclusively by recipients through payroll taxes. States do not contribute to the program. Medicare is called an entitlement program because recipients are entitled to benefits, regardless of assets and income, by paying into the program during their working years. Medicare offers no custodial care services other than those directly connected to skilled or rehabilitative care, and then only for short periods of time.

Medicaid is also a health insurance program, but, as we have mentioned, it is reserved for those who are financially needy. It is a partnership between states and the federal government.

▼ N O T E S   Medicaid is similar to Medicare in the types of health care services it covers, with one significant difference: Medicaid will pay for custodial (non-skilled) care, but primarily in a skilled nursing facility.

Covered services

States are required to cover at least the following services as part of their Medicaid programs (some states offer additional benefits):

General medical services

- Physician's services

- Inpatient hospital services (except for tuberculosis or mental diseases)

- Medical and surgical dental services

- Ambulatory services, such as outpatient hospital services and rural health clinic services

- Lab and x-ray services

Long-term care services

- Services in a skilled-nursing facility for those 21 and older

- Transportation to medical facilities, via taxi or other commercial transportation provider with which your state may contract

- Limited home health care services (see page 81)

Medicaid and home health care

Medicaid does, in limited instances, cover a portion of the cost of custodial care at home under a federal Home and Community-Based Services (HCBS) waiver or the PACE program (Program of All-Inclusive Care for the Elderly). The HCBS program is focused on attempting to keep younger individuals with intellectual and developmental disabilities in the community. PACE focuses on frail elderly people. Both are designed to give states flexibility to develop programs that keep people at home longer rather than institutionalize them at what likely would be a greater expense.

In order to qualify, patients generally have to show that their health or cognitive skills have declined so severely that nursing home placement is imminent. Eligibility is restricted to those with limited assets and income. These programs are not available to people with retirement portfolios or income sufficient to support a middle-class lifestyle.

There is one other issue to consider. States exercise stringent cost containment procedures because of the fear of abuse. This results in caps on enrollments and resulting long waits. The problem is best summed up in a 2000 report[1] from the National Health Law Program, which found that states use the waiver program cautiously for fear that family caregivers will figuratively come out of the woodwork and ask the state to pay for services they themselves are providing for free. They fear that the result of that would be that rather than save money, the program would actually cost more than nursing-home care.

---

[1] *Addressing Home and Community-Based Waiver Waiting Lists Through the Medicaid Program,* by Jane Perkins and Manju Kulkarni for the National Health Law Program, May 20, 2000.

▼ N O T E S In my experience, very few of my clients received home health care benefits or funding for assisted living through either the HCBS or PACE programs. Any attorney fluent in Medicaid funding will tell you as much.

Qualifying for Medicaid

Medical eligibility

Medical eligibility may vary somewhat, as some states impose slightly different conditions, but in general, the applicant is eligible for coverage of custodial care under Medicaid if he or she:

- is unable to perform at least two activities of daily living: bathing, eating, dressing, toileting, continence, and transferring (not being able to get from one point to another without considerable effort); or

- has a severe cognitive disorder requiring constant supervision.

Eligibility for benefits has been substantially affected by the Deficit Reduction Act of 2005, which was signed into law by president Bush on February 8th, 2006. The changes in eligibility, described below, should be carefully reviewed.

The following is a general discussion of how someone qualifies for Medicaid benefits. Remember, rules vary by state and often change.

Financial eligibility

There are two financial criteria considered when qualifying for Medicaid: assets and income. We'll focus first on how individuals qualify and then couples.

Assets

If you apply for Medicaid, the program will divide your assets into three classes:

- *Countable assets* (called *non-exempt* assets in some states)

- *Non-countable assets* (called *exempt* assets in some states)

- *Inaccessible assets*

Countable assets are used to determine Medicaid eligibility. If your assets exceed set limits, they must be *spent down*—used for the Medicaid applicant's care or other legitimate expenses such as food and shelter before you can qualify for benefits. Countable assets are any personal financial resources owned or controlled by the applicant and generally include:

- Cash

- Stocks

- Bonds

- Other investments

- All tax-qualified investments such as those in 401(k), 403(b) or IRA plans.

- Deferred annuities (non-tax or taxed), if not annuitized.

- The cash surrender value on permanent insurance if the death benefit exceeds $1,500. For example, if you own a policy with a death benefit of $50,000, and the cash surrender value grows to $10,000 while you are paying premiums, the cash surrender value is considered a countable asset.

- Vacation property

- Investment property (some states will allow the applicant to keep the property if it generates a certain minimum return).

Non-countable assets are not used to determine eligibility; they are what you are allowed to keep. Non-countable assets are financial resources acknowledged by Medicaid, but they are not used to determine eligibility. Non-countable assets generally include:

- A small sum of money, usually under $3,000.

- A primary residence. However, under the Deficit Reduction Act of 2005 (DRA '05) your state has the right to refuse benefits if the equity in your house is greater than either $500,000 or $750,000, depending on the state.

- Your state is likely to place a lien on the property unless the family meets certain rules. For more information about these exceptions and details on Medicaid crisis planning, see page 103.

- A prepaid funeral (some states limit how much money can be spent).

- Term life insurance

- Business assets, if the applicant derives livelihood from them.

- A car for personal use (some states cap its value).

- Personal items

Inaccessible assets are assets that would have been counted toward eligibility, but they are no longer owned or controlled by the person applying for coverage. There are two ways to make assets inaccessible and therefore protect them from being spent on care: put them in a trust or give them away outright. This strategy is called *Medicaid planning* and is subject to the look-back period.

The look-back period

The *look-back period* is a span of time which a state Medicaid program examines for financial transactions, to see if the applicant made gifts to reduce his assets sufficiently to qualify for benefits. On February 8, 2006, the look-back period was fixed at a uniform five years.[2] Transfers for less than adequate consideration (gifts to family members or transfers into or out of a trust) trigger a period of ineligibility for benefits based on the amount of the transfer and commencing on the date of application for benefits. In every state, this period equals the value of the assets transferred divided by the average monthly cost of nursing home care for a semiprivate room in that state.

Example:

> Massachusetts sets the rate in 2007 at $7,680 a month. If you gift $76,800, you create a ten-month ineligibility for benefits. The ineligibility begins not at the time the gift is made, but when you apply for benefits. In this example, if the application date is April 1st, 2007, you have to wait until February 1st, 2008 to receive Medicaid.

---

2 Previously, the look-back period was three or five years, depending on the nature of the property transfer.

▼ N O T E S **How a couple's assets are treated**

Generally, a married couple's countable assets are considered jointly owned regardless of whose name they are in. Some states, however, allow the *community spouse* (the spouse who does not require long-term care) to keep his or her qualified funds (401(k), 403(b) or IRA). Check with your state for specifics.

Here's an example:

> Before Mary is married, her grandmother gives her stock worth $50,000, which Mary decides to keep in her own name after she gets married. If her spouse applies for Medicaid coverage, the stock will be considered jointly owned, even though she can show that her spouse had nothing to do with acquiring it.

Community spouse resource allowance (CSRA)

The *community spouse resource allowance (CSRA)* is the amount of money the community spouse is allowed to keep when determining Medicaid eligibility. States allow the community spouse to keep a minimum amount of assets. Generally, countable assets of both spouses are added together and then divided by two. The community spouse keeps one half but no less than a *floor* of $20,328 and no more than a *ceiling* of $101,640 (in 2007). These amounts are adjusted yearly.

Your state has the right to raise the $20,328 floor to any amount up to the ceiling of $101,640. California, Florida and Massachusetts, among others, have raised the floor to $101,640. In those states, if a couple has $80,000, the community spouse keeps that amount, rather than just one half.

Here's how the community spouse resource allowance works with a floor of $20,328:

Total assets	The community spouse keeps
$30,000	$20,328
$80,000	$40,000
$400,000	$101,640

Prenuptial agreements

States do not recognize prenuptial agreements when determining Medicaid eligibility. The community spouse's assets are considered countable even if there is a prenuptial agreement that says the assets belong to the community spouse and shall not be claimed by the other. This also applies if the institutional spouse never contributed to the assets, which is common, for example, in second marriages.

Here's an example:

> Craig and Janet (both widowed) decide to marry. Prior to their wedding, they sign a prenuptial agreement to define what would happen to their separate holdings in the event of a divorce or the death of either. They draft wills to make sure that their children receive their due inheritance. Janet enters into the marriage with more than $500,000 from the sale of her deceased husband's business. Craig brings his home and $220,000 into the marriage.

> Three years after they marry, Craig suffers a serious stroke, leaving him paralyzed. After several years of trying to care for him at home, Janet places her husband in a nursing home on February 2007. Their combined assets on that date totaled $720,000, not including their house: Medicaid does not include equity in a home in determining the CSRA.

To qualify for Medicaid coverage, the couple must spend down their combined assets to the Medicaid ceiling, $101,640. Craig will be permitted to keep about $2,000 (the exact amount varies by state) and other non-countable assets. Medicaid will not recognize the prenuptial agreement.

Income

The second financial criterion that Medicaid considers is income. The following explains how the program treats income if either single or married.

How an individual's income is treated

Medicaid considers all income of its applicants, regardless of how it is earned, available to be spent on care.

There are two exceptions to this rule. A Medicaid recipient is allowed to keep:

- A small personal-needs allowance (usually between $30 and $82 per month) to pay for items like clothing, toiletries and medical expenses not covered by Medicare or Medicaid

- The amounts needed to pay for Medicare Part B and Medicare supplement insurance premiums

Cap states

In approximately half of the states, it does not matter how much your income is, as long as it is less than the private cost of care. A Medicaid recipient simply pays his income, less the deductions above, to the facility. Medicaid makes up the shortfall, on the basis of its reimbursement schedule.

The states that don't follow the above arrangement are called *cap states*. You can qualify for Medicaid but only if your monthly income is less than the cap, which in 2007 is $1,869. The amount is adjusted yearly. If your monthly income exceeds the cap, even by one penny, Medicaid will not pay for nursing home care. In these cases, a special type of trust, called a *Miller trust*, can be established to help the care recipient qualify for Medicaid.

The cap states are:

- Alabama
- Alaska
- Arizona
- Arkansas
- Colorado
- Delaware
- Florida
- Idaho
- Iowa
- Louisiana
- Mississippi
- Nevada
- New Mexico
- Oklahoma
- Oregon
- South Carolina
- South Dakota
- Texas
- Wyoming

Miller trusts

A *Miller trust* has one purpose— to qualify an individual for Medicaid if his or income exceeds the cap. Monthly income is deposited into the trust for the benefit of the Medicaid recipient, who is the trust's beneficiary. The trustee, once a month, issues a check to the individual's nursing home in an amount less than the monthly cap. The balance (the difference between monthly income and the cap) continues to accumulate inside the trust. Upon the care recipient's death, those funds are paid to the state as partial repayment for care.

▼ N O T E S   Example:

> In 2007, Howard requested Medicaid assistance for nursing home care in Florida, a cap state. His monthly income is $1,969, an amount that is $100 over the $1,869 cap. He establishes a Miller trust naming his brother, Stanley, as the trustee. Stanley is instructed to take Howard's monthly income of $1,969 and deposit it into the trust. Each month, Stanley pays the nursing home the cap amount from the trust account. Two years later, Howard dies. The $2,400 that has accumulated over that period plus any interest is paid to the state.

Miller trusts are complicated. If this seems like an option that might work for your family, be sure to consult with an experienced elder-law attorney to find out more (see page 105).

How a couple's income is treated

Unlike assets, a couple's income is not considered joint. With one exception, states do not look at the income of the community spouse (the one who does not require long-term care) when determining eligibility for the spouse applying for Medicaid. The exception is New York, which requires the community spouse to direct a percentage of his or her monthly income, if it exceeds a set amount, toward the care of the spouse who needs Medicaid assistance.

Minimum monthly maintenance needs allowance (MMMNA)

Many community spouses have little income. Therefore, the federal government has attempted to ensure they have a minimum to live on. The spouse is allowed to keep a *minimum monthly maintenance needs allowance (MMMNA)*. The parameters are similar to the floor and ceiling asset amounts a community spouse can keep. In 2007, the minimum income is $1,650 per month. The maximum is $2,541.

What happens if a community spouse's income is less than the MMMNA? In this situation, the individual can make up the difference by drawing from the institutionalized spouse's monthly income. This is referred to as the *income-first rule*.

Here's how it works:

> Sarah's husband, Edward, has recently been admitted to a nursing home. They have $303,640 in assets. They do not own a home. Sarah's Social Security income is $650 a month. Edward receives a pension and Social Security benefits that amount to $3,000 per month. According to Medicaid eligibility rules in every state, Sarah can keep no more than $101,640 asset ceiling and her husband's cash allowance, which in their state is $2,000 for a total of $103,640. Sarah must then spend down $200,000 on nursing home care before her husband can receive Medicaid benefits.

> At this point, Sarah is allowed to keep $1,000 of Edward's monthly income because her $650 monthly income is below the minimum allowance of $1,650. If Sarah can prove to Medicaid that her housing expenses are higher than normal, the amount of income she is allowed to keep may be increased.

> Aside from a small amount for personal expenses, Edward must spend the rest of his pension and Social Security income ($2,000 per month) on his own care.

▼ N O T E S   The website ElderLawAnswers,[3] created by elder-law attorney Harry Margolis, includes calculators that determine Medicaid income allowances for community spouses.

The Deficit Reduction Act of 2005 (DRA '05)

The Deficit Reduction Act of 2005 was signed into law by President Bush on February 8, 2006. Its further restriction of access to Medicaid was a response to repeated abuse of the system by middle-class and, at times, wealthy individuals to qualify for long-term care services, primarily in skilled nursing homes. Here are the major provisions of the bill and their consequences:

- The look-back period was increased to five years for all transfers.

- Ineligibility from Medicaid benefits now begins on the date of application for Medicaid assistance, and not on the date of the gift. That means any gift during a five year look-back period cannot be protected.

- The income-first rule has become the only means of bringing a community spouse up to the state MMMNA: the couple must first spend down the excess of assets the couple has, and then use the applicant's monthly income to make up the shortfall (review the MMMNA rules on page 90). This devastates couples with assets in excess of $101,640.

- *"Medicaid-friendly" annuities* (see page 101) have been effectively rendered useless. Hundreds of insurance agents, many in partnerships with attorneys, have promoted the use of these instruments. DRA '05 still

---

3   http://www.ElderLawAnswers.com

allows their use, but the state, not the applicant's children, must now be named first beneficiary.

- Home equity can disqualify you. Single or widowed applicants with home equity exceeding either $500,000 or $750,000 (each state can choose which amount) are disqualified from Medicaid benefits until they spend down to that amount.

- Medicaid now considers deposits in a continuing care retirement community countable assets.

- All states are now able to expand Long-Term Care Partnership benefits to residents (see page 140 for an explanation of this program).

▼ N O T E S **Planning for long-term care _vs_ Medicaid planning**

This book is focused on creating and funding a plan that protects your family and retirement portfolio from the risk of needing care. That goal is accomplished by creating a plan for long-term care.

The goal of qualifying for Medicaid (Medicaid planning) is not to protect a family but to qualify an individual for benefits. Here is an advertisement that confirms that reality:

How to get Medicaid coverage for

NURSING HOME CARE

without selling your house or leaving your family destitute

Most people have heard of Medicaid but few truly understand how it works.

Attend a free workshop on Medicaid Planning presented by an elder-law attorney and learn the following:

- _Protect your hard-earned assets from growing nursing home costs_

- _Protect your most important asset – your family home from the state_

- _Protect an inheritance for you and your children_

Here's another advertisement for a seminar in Florida:

SAY "NO" TO LONG TERM CARE?

FACT: Many people who have purchased long-term care insurance have made a costly mistake. Recent changes in the 1996 Health Insurance Portability and Accountability Act require long-term care policies to meet new eligibility standards.

Many policies prior to HIPA act of 1996 will not qualify for favorable tax treatment or grandfather clause. This is why (name of the company) is having a FREE Eye-OPENING seminar to discuss the following topics...

- *Find out if your existing policy qualifies for favorable tax treatment*

- *Learn how to protect assets from Medicaid spend-down without purchasing nursing-home insurance*

- *Learn what assets are exempt from the Medicaid Spend Down process according to the Kennedy-Kassebaum Health Insurance Reform Bill*

- *How to juggle assets between spouses while living*

- *Learn how to pass assets to children while avoiding the 36/60 look-back trap*

- *Divert income into a Miller trust and protect a spouse at home.*

- *Learn how the Medicaid spend-down process actually works*

- *Perform current asset and income tests on your existing estate to see if you qualify*

- *Should you go through probate? Do you need a will? Do you need a trust?*

▼ N O T E S   The intended audience for these seminars appears to be healthy people. Attorneys and insurance agents will likely promote the use of three Medicaid planning methods: giving assets away, putting them in trust and buying an annuity (see page 101).

If you are considering working with an attorney or agent who conducts seminars such as these, here are some things to remember:

- Since Medicaid's long-term care benefits typically only cover care in a skilled nursing facility, the attorney's advice will focus on nursing-home care. In my more than 20 years of practice, nursing homes have been a last, not a first, choice. Ask the lawyer: "Will Medicaid pay for home care, adult day care or assisted living?"

- Medicaid is not free: Transferring qualified funds (assets held in tax-deferred accounts) creates an immediate tax liability.

- The same analysis applies to assets that have a low cost basis (value at acquisition), such as stocks. If those assets are in your name when you die, their cost basis will be deemed to be their current fair market value. As a result, if they're sold shortly following your death, little or no capital-gains tax will be due. However, if instead those same assets are transferred to your children so you can qualify for Medicaid, the recipients of your gift will be saddled with the original low cost basis, which will create a substantial capital-gains tax liability when the assets are sold.

- If you give your home to your children, you will lose the $250,000 ($500,000 for a couple) in capital-gains exclusion for selling your home. Worse, you will pass on to them the original cost basis in the property, meaning your children will pay a large capital gains tax when they sell it.

Ask the attorney or Medicaid planner:

"What are the tax liabilities created by gifting my assets?"

- Medicaid planning can protect assets; simply give them away at least five years before applying for benefits (see the tax consequences above). Lawyers cannot protect income. If married, it is likely the majority of your income will go for your care. This leaves your spouse at home in a difficult situation financially.

Example:

> Mark and Susan are married. His pension is $5,000 per month; she earns $1,700 from Social Security and a small pension. They have $500,000 in assets and their home is worth $400,000. Mark is diagnosed with early stage Alzheimer's. Since they never planned for this possibility and, having considered long-term care insurance, found it expensive, they now visit an attorney. Here is what they hear for the first time:
>
> Lawyer: *"In order to qualify Mark for Medicaid the two of you will have to gift $400,000 to your children because all Susan can keep is $101,640. Then you have to keep Mark at home for five years."*
>
> > Susan: *"Most of our retirement portfolio is in qualified funds."*

97

▼ N O T E S

Lawyer: *"You will have to pay tax at a rate of 35% plus a state tax of 5%."*

Susan: *"I want to keep my husband home for as long as possible. What will pay for his care at home, or if I need adult day care or assisted living?"*

Lawyer: *"Nothing. Medicaid will only pay for nursing home care."*

Susan: *"What do I get to keep if I place my husband in a nursing home?"*

Lawyer: *"As I've mentioned, $101,640 (in 2007), and only your income; Mark's income will have to go towards the cost of his care in a facility."*

Susan: *"That leaves me with about $100,000 and just over $20,000 per year!"*

Lawyer: *"I can annuitize the $400,000 in your name but that creates its own problems. If Mark's funds are qualified, gifting them to you will cause the same tax issues. And even if you annuitize the assets, you will still lose Mark's monthly income."*

- The Medicaid-planning attorney may also not have discussed that transferring assets to another person may have other unintended consequences. Example:

- Transferring assets to your children who have college-aged children may disqualify your grandchildren from student aid.

- Will you be transferring assets to family members who may not be financially responsible?

- Is your child in a sound marriage? Transferring assets to a married child or grandchild who later becomes divorced could result in half (or more) of the assets' going to the former spouse.

Life estates

Life estates are created when you convey your home to another person (usually a child or children), but keep the right to live there and control what happens to the property during your life. Under tax law, the entire value of the house is included in your estate for tax purposes when you die (even though you didn't legally own it), because you had the use of it. Therefore, even if you gift your house and retain a life estate, it will still receive a stepped-up basis at your death. This sounds like a good solution, but there are a few problems:

- If you decide to sell the house, you may lose your capital-gains exemption of $250,000 ($500,000 for a couple).

- Many states are now placing liens on life estates when the life estate holders qualify for Medicaid. This allows the state to recover benefits paid on Medicaid recipients' behalf from the proceeds of the sale of the house.

Trusts

"I was told a trust would protect my assets."

A trust is simply a legal document created to hold assets. The person who establishes the trust is called a *trustor, donor,* or, when the trust holds real estate, *grantor.* The trust is for the benefit of individuals or institutions who are referred to as *beneficiaries.* A *trustee* administers the trust. If the trustor maintains the right to modify or terminate the trust, it's referred to as *revocable*. If the trustor gives up those rights, the trust is called *irrevocable*.

Revocable trusts

A revocable trust will not protect your assets from being spent on your care. Your state doesn't care who owns the assets (in this case, the trust); it is interested only in who has access to them (you).

Irrevocable trusts

Irrevocable trusts are more complicated. If you set up a trust and name yourself or your spouse as a beneficiary, and give the trustee any power to give you money, your state will assume the trustee will use that power to pay for your care. It is highly unlikely that these types of trusts will work to protect your assets.

There are lawyers who recommend that you establish an income-only irrevocable trust. These trusts limit the powers of the trustee to providing the beneficiary with income from the trust. The trustee has no discretion to give the beneficiary principal. If you do not have access to that principal, and if your asset level is under Medicaid limits, you may be able to qualify for benefits.

Even so, consider the following:

- Trusts cannot hold qualified funds such as IRAs, 401(k) or 403(b) plans. Placing these assets in trust therefore creates an immediate tax.

- Your plan is to stay at home for as long as possible. Medicaid pays little or nothing for such care, which means the trustee will be forced to pay for it.

- Even if taxes are not an issue, consider, if you are married, the income problem discussed on page 90.

"Medicaid-friendly" annuities

An *annuity* is an investment in the form of a contract between an investor and another party (usually an insurance company). After placing money into an annuity, the investor receives periodic payments during the life of the contract.

An *immediate annuity* begins payments as soon as funds are invested. Such annuities are used in Medicaid planning because they convert countable assets into an income stream. The income goes toward nursing-home costs, and Medicaid makes up the balance. The annuity's beneficiaries, usually children of the annuity owner, may end up getting the balance of the annuity if the owner dies before exhausting the monthly benefit.

The whole point of the Medicaid annuity is to try to leave money to the annuity owner's children. The Deficit Reduction Act of 2005 (DRA '05) includes a provision mandating that the state, rather than the owner's children or other individuals, be named beneficiary. This effectively eliminates any incentive to purchase the annuity for Medicaid planning purposes.

Estate recovery

All states have the right to recover Medicaid benefits from assets that their recipients either own or control at their death. Until 1993, few states made the effort to recover these assets. Through the Omnibus Budget Reconciliation Act of 1993 (OBRA '93), Congress prodded states to do so. Current efforts are inconsistent, but the trend is clearly moving toward greater recovery of assets. Here are the results of these efforts thus far:

- Many states will now place a lien on a Medicaid recipient's home, even if his spouse still resides there. The lien remains after the Medicaid recipient's death to be repaid when the community spouse dies. The thinking is that the state should not subsidize a child's inheritance.

- States are looking into legislation that will mandate that insurance companies notify Medicaid before they pay a life insurance claim, to determine if the deceased was receiving benefits.

Illegal gifts

- Some states, Connecticut in particular, are putting families on notice that if they receive gifts of money during the look-back period, the person who receives the money could be liable. Connecticut's Transferee Liability Law went into effect July 6, 2005, and has all but halted efforts to protect assets.

- Iowa now has a law providing that if an individual transfers assets to someone and then files a Medicaid application within five years (regardless of the penalty period triggered by the transfers), the state can recover from the transferee the lesser of the full amount paid by the state for the Medicaid patient's care or the value of the gifts made by the Medicaid recipient.

- Approximately thirty states have so-called *filial support laws* that seek to hold children responsible for paying their parents' long-term care costs. Although the federal government has stated that such laws are illegal, many states are looking for ways to overcome the objections.

- Many states are requesting permission from the federal government to increase the look-back period for outright gifts to six years and for transfers into or out of a trust to ten years.

Still want to apply for Medicaid?

It is critical that you understand the financial consequences of relying on Medicaid. Look carefully at the advertisements earlier in this section. Was there one word about any of the issues we just covered or the emotional and physical consequences to which your family will be subjected all the years you may be at home? In all my years in practice, families have come to see me when most of this damage had already taken place.

In short, Medicaid planning is counterproductive to a plan to protect the emotional and physical wellbeing of a family and the retirement portfolio on which it will depend.

Medicaid planning in a crisis

Some professionals in the long-term care insurance industry believe Medicaid should never be used when a person has any assets or a home. That is too simplistic a view. There are some situations in which Medicaid benefits may be appropriate. In the following examples, taking steps to preserve money isn't Medicaid planning in its conventional sense, but a matter of applying Medicaid regulations to avoid the total impoverishment of the program's intended beneficiaries—people in the beginning stages of a chronic illness, or already sick individuals who need or are receiving nursing-home care but can no longer afford to pay for it. Here are some ideas:

▼ N O T E S **Protecting a small business**

If a Medicaid applicant derives a livelihood from certain assets, such as a business, most, if not all, states will let that applicant keep those assets temporarily. Since it is unlikely that someone who needs nursing-home care will qualify for this exception, it appears this approach has little purpose.

However, on more than one occasion I have been able to protect a business for a community spouse by simply transferring it to her. Any assets used in generating income are exempt. The income, now earned by the community spouse, is never counted in determining the institutionalized spouse's Medicaid benefits.

If you have a disabled child: the supplemental-needs trust (SNT)

Assets that might otherwise have to be spent on your long-term care can be protected if you have a disabled child. Federal law allows assets to be transferred outright to a child who is disabled under Social Security disability standards. The assets can also be gifted into a *supplemental-needs trust (SNT)*. This rule is indispensable in protecting children with special needs. If this applies to you, I strongly recommended that you seek out an attorney who understands the law.

Protecting a primary residence

Prior to DRA '05, a primary home was a non-countable asset: Medicaid did not count its value among an applicant's assets. However, DRA '05 has introduced new rules for the treatment of Medicaid applicants' homes. The law mandates that Medicaid deny benefits to applicants with homes in which they have more than $500,000 in equity (the states can raise this to $750,000). This law is aimed at individuals who attempt to qualify for Medicaid by sheltering assets in expensive homes.

Aside from this, a primary residence can be gifted to:

- a spouse;

- a child who is disabled, blind or under 21;

- a child who lived with the parent now applying for Medicaid, if it can be shown that the child has resided there for at least two years and provided care.

- Many states will allow the residence to be transferred to a sibling who has lived there for at least one year and has an equity interest.

Choosing a lawyer

If you are considering applying for Medicaid, my advice is to work closely with a lawyer. The practice of Medicaid law is a specialized field and few lawyers can speak its language fluently. Here are some suggestions for finding an attorney with expertise in this field:

- Speak to the social worker at a local hospital. Many have dealt with nursing home placement and are familiar with attorneys who work in the field.

- Speak to your doctor, but ensure he has worked on Medicaid issues with the attorney he recommends.

- Local support groups such as ones for Alzheimer's, Parkinson's and stroke victims and their families are an excellent source when you're looking for an experienced attorney. Ask your local hospital for these groups' contact information.

- If there is a lawyer in your family, ask him or her to find a lawyer who specializes in elder law.

- Visit the website ElderLawAnswers,[4] which offers comprehensive information on elder-law issues and provides referrals to attorneys who specialize in this area.

Interviewing a lawyer

Once you've found a good candidate, be sure to ask these questions to assess the lawyer's competence in Medicaid law:

- Has the attorney ever spoken or written about Medicaid and Medicaid planning?

- How does the attorney charge, and what specific work is performed? Ensure the attorney is willing to write you a comprehensive follow-up letter after your initial meeting. It is difficult to absorb everything a lawyer says in a first meeting. The letter will clarify the information discussed.

- Has the attorney ever worked in tandem with a financial planner to establish a client's long-term care plan?

The majority of attorneys who understand how long-term care is financed use Medicaid responsibly to help families in a crisis. In an informal survey, those attorneys generally agree that, with few exceptions, clients came to see them because their family has never had a discussion about the consequences that needing care would have on caregivers and retirement portfolios.

---

4 http://www.ElderLawAnswers.com

Understanding Long-Term Care Insurance **6**

"Why do I need long-term care insurance?" 110

A brief history of long-term care insurance 115

How policies work 117

Basic policy parameters 117

    Daily benefit (benefit level) 117

    Benefit period 117

    Pool of funds 117

How policies pay 118

    Reimbursement 118

    Indemnity 118

    Cash benefit 119

Policy formats 119

    Facility care only 119

    Home health care only 120

    Comprehensive care 120

Standard policy language 121

    30-day free look 121

    Guaranteed renewability 121

    No prior hospitalization 121

    Outlines of standard coverage 121

    Specific exclusions 122

    Unintentional-lapse provision 122

    Benefit triggers 122

        Inability to perform activities of daily living 122

        Cognitive impairment 123

        Medical necessity 123

    Elimination period 123

    Bed reservation 124

107

Alternate plan of care 124

Home modification.. 124

Care coordination 124

Respite care 125

Waiver of premium 125

Optional policy provisions 125

Restoration of benefits.. 125

Survivorship option 126

Accelerated-payment (limited-pay, paid-up) option 126

Nonforfeiture 126

Return-of-premium option 127

Inflation protection 127

Tax-qualified long-term care insurance 127

Criteria of tax-qualified plans 128

Non-tax-qualified policies 129

Should you consider a non-tax-qualified policy? 129

Taxation of benefits of tax-qualified policies.. 130

Deducting the premiums on tax-qualified policies 130

Individual policyholders 130

Eligible premium 131

Non-self-employed individual policyholders 131

Self-employed individuals (sole proprietors)................................ 132

Premiums paid for parents' policies 133

Partnerships.. 134

S corporations 135

Limited-liability companies (LLC)... 136

Professional corporations (PC).. 137

C corporations 137

State tax incentives 138

Employer-sponsored policies 138

True group 138

Affinity group 138

Multi-life... 139

Federal Long-Term Care Insurance Program 139

Long-Term Care Partnership programs 140

Current protection methods.. 140

    California and Connecticut: dollar-for-dollar asset protection.................... 140

    New York: unlimited asset protection.. 141

    Indiana: hybrid asset protection 141

    Massachusetts: selective asset protection.. 141

Partnership programs: advantages and disadvantages................................... 141

Paying for a long-term care policy... 142

    Funding from an IRA... 143

    Reverse mortgages (Home Equity Conversion Mortgages, HECMs) 143

    Life settlements 145

Children contributing to the cost... 145

▼ N O T E S   First, a disclaimer: I am a proponent of long-term care insurance. I believe it is the best way to fund a long-term care plan, if you can afford the premium. It is unreasonable to assume that any government program will pay for the type of care you or your loved one might need where you want it most — at home.

A 2003 *Consumer Reports* article[1] says essentially the same thing:

> *"...few people are able to amass such sums and the government is unlikely to pick up the tab. The only obvious answer is long-term-care insurance."*

"Why do I need long-term care insurance?"

A quick review may be helpful to overcome any last doubts you may have about the importance of this type of coverage. Let's do it in a question-and-answer format:

> *"What if I don't live a long life or even if I do, never get sick and need care? Wouldn't buying a policy be a waste of money?*

I am going to agree with you; you may not live a long life and even if you do, you may never become frail and need care. You likely think that people who purchase long-term care insurance believe these things will happen. However, most don't.

They believe, as you likely do, that the worst things in life will happen to someone else; few live their lives in fear. So, even though the policyholder believes he will not need care, he understands that if he does, taking care of him over a period of years could have severe consequences for his family and retirement portfolio.

---

1 "Do you need long-term care insurance?", *Consumer Reports,* December 2003

Consider the similarity to life insurance: the risk of dying during one's working years is statistically very low (less than 2%). Yet people who love their family understand that even though the risk is insignificant, the consequences to their family and assets would be catastrophic. Here, the reasoning is reduced to a simple formula:

- Low risk of dying during working years x (huge consequences to your family + the need to plan to protect your family) = the need to purchase life insurance.

It's exactly the same reason people purchase long-term care insurance:

- Low risk of needing care x (huge consequences to your family + the need to plan to protect your family) = the need to purchase long-term care insurance.

People purchase long-term care insurance for the same reason they buy life insurance: they love their family. They know the policy will allow their spouse and children to supervise care, and not to have to provide it.

"I really do believe I have enough assets to pay for the cost of care if I need it."

Many people believe that long-term care insurance protects assets. It does, but only indirectly. It primarily protects income. Retirees live on income generated by Social Security, pensions and the draw-down on their qualified funds, such as IRAs, 401(k) or 403(b) plans. Other investments, such as stocks and bonds outside qualified funds, as well as the income earned on them, are generally not used to support their needs because they want a cushion should something happen in the future.

People have passions in life such as horses, golf, travel and fishing. Collectively, they amount to a lifestyle. A retirement portfolio generates the income necessary to support both a person's lifestyle and his continuing commitments to his family and community.

If you or someone you love needs custodial care over a period of years, you now understand that no federal or state program will pay for it (Medicaid being an exception, but almost exclusively for care in a nursing home). Also consider what in your retirement portfolio has been allocated to pay for your care. If you're like most people in this regard, the answer is *nothing*.

Here's the irony: since nothing has been allocated, in reality all of it will be allocated to pay for care. Where else can the money come from?

Long-term care insurance protects income by paying for care that otherwise will have to be purchased at the expense of your family's lifestyle. It therefore allows your family to continue to live the lifestyle to which they've become accustomed. Without insurance, your lifestyle—and theirs—may be severely impacted. At worst, you may have to start liquidating your invest-ments. This is not merely a hypothetical possibility; I have seen it over and over again in my practice.

If something in life is important to you or a loved one, you need to protect it. Protecting a long-term care plan with long-term care insurance can help you do that.

"I have almost $2 million. I've read in **Consumer Reports** *that I can easily self-insure the cost of care."*

That may be true. In fact, for years I told those of my clients who were wealthy that they could easily pay the cost of care. I was politely chastised by a number of them who were going to purchase long-term care insurance despite my opinion. Here's what they taught me:

- Many had a prior experience with long-term care and saw first-hand what the failure to have a plan did to their family and finances.

- Not one of them believed that they would get frail and need care over a long period of time. However, they now understood what failure to plan would do to their family and finances.

- They also understood that care is very expensive.

- They added the two sets consequences, those to their family and finances, together and concluded that purchasing long-term care insurance is a prudent and cost-effective way to protect both their loved ones as well as their portfolios.

In my opinion, *Consumer Reports* failed to address some other issues:

- Paying for care from qualified funds creates an immediate tax liability.

- If you have to liquidate assets with a low cost basis to pay for care, you will be subject to capital-gains tax.

Consumer Reports seems to suggest that those with modest assets consider Medicaid as part of a plan for financing care. Here are some problems with that strategy:

- As mentioned, there may be serious tax implications to cashing in certain types of assets.

- Once an institutionalized spouse qualifies for benefits, the majority of his or her monthly income likely will have to be applied towards the cost of care. In my experience, the community spouse will have little monthly income and likely will have to rely on children for support.

In short, *Consumer Reports* appears not to understand that long-term care insurance is part of an overall plan to protect not the policyholder, but his family and lifestyle.

"But I was told by my financial advisor that it's a waste of money."

Many advisors will tell clients with substantial assets that they don't need long-term care insurance. I don't believe it is the right advice. Consider this story:

> One of my clients had a mother who was diagnosed with Alzheimer's at age 67. The family was very wealthy and had been told by their lawyer, accountant and financial advisor that the parents could easily pay for care out-of-pocket. I reviewed the portfolio and concluded that this was a fair assessment—it was unlikely the principal of the family's assets would ever be used, let alone lost, to pay for the mother's care.

Yet, the client had come to me to find out how she could get her mother to qualify for Medicaid. *"Rationally, we understand trying to qualify for Medicaid seems inappropriate,"* she said, *"but the illness is running our lives. We don't know what to do, and we are still afraid that there won't be enough money."*

Years later, the family called me. They said their father died before their mother, and they believe the stress of caring for his wife contributed to his death. They told me he was always worrying about money, even though they reassured him there was enough.

Long-term care insurance would have provided an important psychological benefit: the family would have been assured that they would likely never run out of funds (even though intellectually they knew it was not going to happen). Postscript to the story: The client purchased long-term care insurance for himself despite the recommendation of his advisor.

A brief history of long-term care insurance

Long-term care insurance is a relatively new product. Early policies (issued between 1975 and 1993) were commonly known as *nursing-home insurance.* Many policies had limitations and hard-to-understand language.

The long-term care insurance policies available today are far more sophisticated. Insurance companies now offer flexible options to meet the needs and budgets of a wide variety of people. They are very effective in providing funding for the full continuum of care, not just nursing homes.

▼ N O T E S   To understand long-term care insurance as it exists today, it's helpful to look at its evolution over the past 20 years, since policies have changed dramatically. Here are some key differences between most early policies and those sold today:

Early policies (up to about 1993)	Today's policies
May not have covered Alzheimer's.	Cover Alzheimer's disease and related dementia.
Required a prior hospitalization for benefits to start.	No prior hospital stay is necessary.
Required skilled care to be received before non-skilled care benefits commenced.	Do not require a prior need for skilled care before custodial-care benefits commence.
Policies could be cancelled after a claim.	Policies are *guaranteed renewable:* the insurance company must unconditionally renew your policy so long as you continue to pay your premium.
Generally only covered skilled home care.	Cover custodial care and skilled care.
Required a prior nursing-home stay before benefits commenced.	Do not require a prior nursing-home stay for benefits to commence.
Policy language was unclear and vague.	Policy triggers and benefits are clearly detailed.
There were no state or federal government standards.	National Association of Insurance Commissioners (NAIC)-developed coverage standards in most states.

How policies work

Every long-term care insurance company offers various coverage options, but generally, a long-term care insurance policy will pay out benefits for care received at home, adult day-care centers, room and board at assisted-living facilities (if the policyholder requires assistance with activities of daily living or suffers from cognitive impairment), and care provided in nursing homes.

Basic policy parameters

Three basic parameters control the size of a policy's benefit and the length of time over which it will pay:

Daily benefit (benefit level)

The *daily benefit* or *benefit level* is the maximum amount of money the insurance company will pay for long-term care services on a daily basis. The higher the daily benefit, the more expensive the long-term care insurance policy becomes. Benefit levels generally range from $40 to $500, and sometimes more, per day.

Benefit period

This is the period of time the benefit payments last after payment has started. Options generally range from one year to lifetime.

Pool of funds

Most insurance companies pay benefits from a *pool of funds*. Its size is determined by multiplying the daily benefit by the length of the benefit period in years.

▼ NOTES   The pool of funds permits the effective benefit period to
be lengthened whenever the maximum daily benefit is not
drawn, as usually occurs in reimbursement policies. It's a good
idea to make sure the insurance companies you're considering
offer this approach.

For example:

> The purchase of a $100 daily benefit for five years re-
> sults in a $182,625 pool of funds ($100 per day *x* 5 years
> *x* 365.25 days per year). If you draw less than $100 per
> day, you will be able to use the policy for more than its
> nominal five-year benefit period.

How policies pay

There are three ways insurance companies pay benefits on
long-term care insurance policies: *reimbursement, indemnity* or
cash benefit.

Reimbursement

The holder of a reimbursement-based policy must submit
bills to the insurance company for care covered in the insurance contract. The insurance company then reimburses either
the policyholder or the care provider directly, for actual care
expenses, up to the maximum daily benefit purchased.

Indemnity

An indemnity policy pays out the entire daily benefit, regardless of actual expenses, as long as the policyholder shows he
received at least one service per day for which the insurance
company will pay.

For example: A home care visit for one hour a day, received by the holder of a policy that covers home care, would result in the payment of the maximum daily benefit purchased. The policyholder keeps the difference between the daily benefit and the actual cost of care.

Cash benefit

A cash benefit pays the entire daily benefit without requiring the policyholder to show proof of care. This is the least restrictive, and most expensive, option.

Policy formats

Long-term care insurance policies can be purchased in one of three formats: *facility care only, home health care only* or *comprehensive care.* Your family's specific needs should dictate your choice of policy format.

Facility care only

As the name implies, facility-care-only policies cover only long-term care that is provided in settings such as nursing homes and assisted-living facilities. These policies are less expensive than others, but remember that you may want to receive care at home, and this type of policy will not pay for it.

Advantage:

- May make sense if you are in a rural area where it would be difficult to get home care services.

Disadvantage:

- Your situation may change. What if you move to a place where home care is feasible? What if you decide to move in with your daughter and you'd like to compensate her for her help.

Home health care only

This format pays only for home care and adult day care. Insurance companies report that the majority of their claims are being paid for home care.

Advantage:

- If you have the family infrastructure that can help you stay at home, this format may make sense.

Disadvantage:

- Like a facility-only policy, a home-health-care-only policy may not be what's needed if circumstances change over time. What if you or your family wants to move you to an assisted-living facility, or your care needs become so complex that you need nursing-home care?

Comprehensive care

By far, most long-term care insurance policies sold today are comprehensive care policies. They cover a full range of care services, whether provided in the home, a nursing home, an assisted-living facility or in adult day care. The benefit of these policies is clear from their name—they are comprehensive. They pay for all the different types of care that people may need as they age and as their illnesses progress. Although few people want or need nursing home care, it is still part of the continuum of care, and ultimately, some people will require it. Some can be cared for safely only in skilled nursing facilities.

Standard policy language

All policies issued since 1993 are controlled by regulations developed by the National Association of Insurance Commissioners (NAIC). The following terms are standard in all policies:

30-day free look

After you purchase a long-term care insurance policy, you have thirty days to review it. You can cancel your policy at any time during this period at no cost to you.

Guaranteed renewability

As long as premiums are paid when they are due, the insurance company cannot cancel the policy, even after the insured has received benefits and subsequently gets better.

No prior hospitalization

All states prohibit long-term care policies from requiring a prior hospital stay before they will begin paying benefits.

Outlines of standard coverage

To encourage consumer awareness, most states require insurance companies, through their agents and representatives, to give prospective buyers outlines of their long-term care insurance coverage, before they apply for insurance. These outlines typically summarize key policy provisions, including benefit levels, restrictions, policy renewal guidelines and pre-existing conditions. Most states require these outlines to be written in a manner that is easily understood by the average consumer.

▼ NOTES **Specific exclusions**

Most states allow insurance companies to use standard exclusions to help reduce their risk exposure. For example, insurance companies usually don't cover care that is needed because of alcoholism and substance abuse. While policies now must cover Alzheimer's disease and other *organic cognitive disabilities* (disabilities that result from changes to the structure of the brain), they are usually not required to cover nonorganic mental disorders such as schizophrenia. Some states, however, require long-term care policies to cover all mental conditions, regardless of their origin, and some companies offer this coverage even when it is not required. Self-inflicted injuries and illnesses resulting from acts of war are also generally not covered. Be sure to check your policy carefully.

Unintentional-lapse provision

This provision allows policy owners who miss a premium payment to reinstate the policy up to six months later, if the lapse was due to a cognitive or physical impairment.

Benefit triggers

Benefit triggers are events that must take place before long-term care policy benefits are paid. They include:

Inability to perform activities of daily living

This is an inability to perform without substantial assistance two or more activities of daily living (ADLs): toileting, bathing, dressing, eating, transferring (getting from one point to another without falling) or continence (see page 30).

Cognitive impairment

A cognitive impairment, which can include problems with memory, perception, problem-solving, and conceptualization, can trigger benefits if it leads to a requirement for substantial assistance.

Medical necessity

A medically necessary service is one that:

- is in accordance with accepted standards of medical practice for the diagnosis and treatment of the policy-holder's condition;

- is delivered in the least restrictive health care setting required by his condition, when possible;

- is not given solely for the patient's convenience or that of his family or health care provider (in other words, the service must be essential).

Some policies written before January 1, 1997 included a medical trigger, which was eliminated by the Health Insurance Portability and Accountability Act of 1996 (HIPAA). All tax-qualified policies (see page 127) issued in 1997 or later can have only ADL and cognitive impairment benefit triggers.

Elimination period

The *elimination period,* sometimes called the *waiting period,* is the period of time that must elapse between a benefit trigger and the day coverage starts. Elimination periods generally range from zero days to one year (some states will not permit more than 180 days).

There are three types of elimination periods: *calendar, days-of-service* and *hybrid.* These are discussed in detail on page 155.

123

▼ N O T E S **Bed reservation**

Some nursing homes have waiting lists for admission. If a nursing-home resident is hospitalized, his bed is often given to another patient. He may then no longer be able to return to the nursing home when he is discharged from the hospital. The bed reservation feature pays the daily benefit for nursing-home care when you must leave the nursing home to be hospitalized. Bed reservation benefit periods usually range from 20 to 50 days.

Alternate plan of care

Under this provision, also called an *emerging trends benefit,* the carrier agrees to review any type of current care that was not specifically covered when the policy was issued.

Home modification

Every carrier offers you the right to take a lump sum of dollars from your benefit pool to make your home accessible.

Example:

> Joan is diagnosed with osteoporosis and mild dementia. Her family wants to keep her home but needs to invest in ramps for a wheelchair and a handicap-accessible bathroom. The request would be presented to the insurance company, which will probably pay for the modifications, because keeping Joan home would be less expensive for it than placing her in a skilled-nursing facility.

Care coordination

This provision is often overlooked but provides a critical benefit to families. A *care manager* or *care coordinator* can create a care plan based on the patient's illness and the wishes of the family. This can be of great help to children who are busy raising their own families, or do not live close to their parents.

A care coordinator may help choose the best way to receive care—in an assisted-living facility, adult day care center, a nursing home or even a hospice. The care coordinator also helps negotiate prices, coordinate schedules and monitor the care recipient on behalf of family members who don't live nearby.

Respite care

This provision pays for temporary institutional care or alternative home care while the home-based caregiver goes on vacation or takes a break.

Waiver of premium

This provision waives the premium requirement for policyholders who become disabled and are collecting benefits, usually after the elimination period has been met.

Optional policy provisions

Generally referred to as *riders,* the following provisions are usually offered at additional cost:

Restoration of benefits

This provision restores the full benefit period after some benefits have already been paid. To qualify, you usually must have fully recuperated and must not suffer a relapse for a minimum period (usually six months). If you require long-term care within six months of recovering from a prior period of care, full benefits will be restored only if the cause is different from the first illness or injury.

▼ NOTES Unless it is built into the policy, the restoration of benefits provision is not recommended unless you plan on purchasing the product in your thirties or fourties, when there is a possibility you might recover from your disability.

Survivorship option

This benefit applies to couples who purchase long-term care insurance policies together. Typically, if a policy has been paid for over a period of time (usually ten years), and one spouse dies, the surviving spouse's policy is considered *paid-up* and requires no further payments. This can be an important feature, especially when one spouse is older than the other.

Accelerated-payment (limited-pay, paid-up) option

Most insurance companies permit a policyholder to pay for his policy in full over a set period of time, usually ten or twenty years. This option may be attractive to younger, higher-income people who can afford to pay for the policy in a shorter amount of time. Some states don't allow this option at all, or mandate a *nonforfeiture* benefit. That means the policy owner will still have benefits equal to the amount of money he paid toward the policy, if he or she is unable to pay the cost of the policy in full during the limited-pay period.

Nonforfeiture

Nonforfeiture must be offered as an option to all purchasers of tax-qualified long-term care policies. If this option is selected, and the policyholder stops paying the policy premiums after three years, he can elect *paid-up* status for the policy. This means that the policy will remain in force with a reduced maximum benefit, equal to the amount of premiums paid into the policy.

This rider may be worth considering if you are concerned that you might not be able to afford the premium payments in the future. However, the persistency rate on long-term care policies is very high: policyholders typically continue paying their premiums as they come due.

Return-of-premium option

This option provides for a return of the premiums paid for a long-term care policy at the insured's death. The refund is typically reduced by any benefits that had been paid on the policy, but some companies will refund all premiums paid without deducting any paid benefits. The refund can be made payable to the insured's estate or named beneficiary. Return-of-premium options are quite expensive, often almost doubling a policy's premium. It might interest those concerned by the prospect of spending money on a premium but never using the benefits. However, because of its cost, few people actually purchase this feature.

Inflation protection

Inflation protection is critical, since you can expect the cost of long-term care to increase annually. Insurance companies must offer inflation protection as an option on all long-term care policies. There are typically three types of inflation protection. See Chapter 7 for a detailed description and recommendations.

Tax-qualified long-term care insurance

Tax-qualified long-term care insurance policies were created under the Health Insurance Portability and Accountability Act (HIPAA) in 1997. The goal was twofold: First, Congress wanted companies to further standardize long-term care policies so consumers would not be confused when comparing them; and second, they wanted to encourage consumers to purchase long-term care insurance.

Criteria of tax-qualified plans

In order for a long-term care insurance policy to be considered tax-qualified, it must meet certain criteria:

- It cannot have a medical necessity trigger. In other words, policy owners cannot receive benefits for medical needs. This makes sense because health insurance covers medical expenses. Using a long-term care policy to pay for medical costs would only reduce the benefit amount available to cover future nonmedical care and would also increase the chance of future premium increases.

- To receive benefits, the insured person must be certified by a licensed health care practitioner as *chronically ill:* either unable to perform, without substantial assistance, at least two activities of daily living (see page 30) for at least 90 days. This rule does not apply to patients with a cognitive impairment.

  Note that this rule does not mean that the insured has to wait 90 days to draw benefits; he has to wait the policy's elimination period (see page 123).

- If the insured receives a return of any premium or earns dividends (from mutual insurance companies for example), this money can be used only to reduce future long-term care insurance policy premiums or increase the policy's benefits. Any refund or dividend not used for this purpose will be taxed to the extent it was deducted by the policyholder.

- The policy cannot have a cash surrender benefit, nor can the policy be assigned, pledged or borrowed against. In this respect, long-term care insurance differs from life insurance.

- Reimbursement-based tax-qualified policies cannot pay benefits for services covered under Medicare.

Non-tax-qualified policies

Non-tax-qualified long-term care policies can contain a medical-necessity trigger that allows benefits to be paid if the insured requires medical attention. These types of policies do not require the insured to be chronically ill to receive benefits. Policy owners can also qualify for benefits by showing that they need assistance with two or more activities of daily living, or that they require supervision due to a cognitive impairment.

While some insurance companies continue to offer policies that do not meet the requirements for tax benefits, a majority of insurers have now made a commitment to issue only tax-qualified policies.

Should you consider a non-tax-qualified policy?

Generally, no. You may not even find a company that offers one, anyway. In 2005, more than 98% of new policies issued were tax-qualified.[2] It is becoming increasingly more difficult to find the non-qualified variety.

Also, because non-qualified policies make it easier to qualify for benefits, you are more likely to be subjected to premium increases if you buy one.

---

2 *2006 Broker World LTCi Survey*

▼ NOTES **Taxation of benefits of tax-qualified policies**

The benefits of reimbursement-based (see page 118) tax-qualified long-term care policies are tax-free.

The benefits of indemnity policies (see page 118) are tax-free only up to $260 per day (in 2007) or the actual cost of care, whichever is higher.[3]

Deducting the premiums on tax-qualified policies

Individual policyholders

A portion of the premium paid in a tax year for a tax-qualified long-term care policy is called *eligible premium*. That's the most individual taxpayers can deduct, although individuals who are not either self-employed or owners of more than 2% of a partnership, S corporation or LLC, are subject to an additional restriction: only medical expenses, including eligible health and long-term care insurance premiums, in excess of 7.5% of their adjusted gross income may be deducted.

---

3   Internal Revenue Code §7702(a)(2), §7702B(d), §105(b)

Eligible premium

Policyholder age	Deduction for 2007*
40 or younger	$290
41–50	$550
51–60	$1,110
61–70	$2,950
71 or older	$3,680

* Source: IRS. See *Tax Changes for Individuals* (http://www.irs.gov/publications/ p553/ch01.html) or *Tax Guide for Older Americans* (http://www.irs.gov/ publications/p554/ch04.html) for subsequent tax years' eligible premiums.

Non-self-employed individual policyholders

- A non-self-employed individual taxpayer who claims the deduction of eligible long-term care insurance premiums must file an itemized return (IRS Form 1040, Schedule A).

- The eligible premium, based on age (see the above table), is added to all deductible medical expenses such as medical insurance premiums and medical expenses that have not been reimbursed.

- The total of these expenses that exceeds 7.5% of the taxpayer's adjusted gross income (AGI) is deductible from gross income on Schedule A.

Example:

> Peter, a 61-year-old man who is not self employed, purchases a tax-qualified long-term care insurance policy that costs $3,000 a year. For 2007, the eligible portion of that premium for his age is $2,950. His other medical expenses are $2,200 for a total of $5,150. His adjusted gross income (AGI) is $75,000.

AGI $75,000

Maximum insurance premium
eligible for deduction...$2,950

Other eligible medical expenses $2,200

Total eligible medical expenses.............................$5,150

Nondeductible medical expenses
(7.5% of AGI)...$5,625

Deduction
(medical expenses in excess of 7.5% of AGI)..............$0

AGI after medical deduction.............................$75,000

The tax savings from a tax-qualified long-term care insurance policy might be greater if a husband and wife, filing jointly, each purchase a long-term care insurance policy, especially if one of them has little or no income.

Note that individual policyholders who are not self-employed but own more than 2% of partnerships, S corporations or limited-liability companies (LLC), are not subject to this restriction and can deduct the entire eligible premium. See the relevant section for your situation below.

Self-employed individuals (sole proprietors)

The tax code treats self-employed individuals (termed *sole proprietors*) more favorably than individuals who are not self-employed. The sole proprietor:

- can treat his long-term care insurance premium as a *self-employment health insurance premium*.[4]

- must report the premium as income on his individual tax return, but can then deduct it there as self-employment health insurance premium.[5] However, the premium *is* subject to self-employment tax (calculated and filed on Schedule SE).[6]

- can deduct the eligible premiums his business paid for his spouse and tax dependents, such as parents.[7]

- can deduct the actual premiums paid for employees from business income.[8] These premiums are excluded from the employees' income and benefits are tax-free.[9]

- can discriminate: He is not subject to anti-discrimination rules, and can discriminate by class, offering the insurance to some employee classes, but not others.[10]

Premiums paid for parents' policies

Premiums paid for a parent who is a dependent of the child by IRS definition are deductible as qualifying medical expenses.

---

4 Internal Revenue Code §162(l)

5 Internal Revenue Code §162(l), §162(l)(2)(C), §213(d)

6 Internal Revenue Code §162(l)(4)

7 Internal Revenue Code §162(l), §162(l)(2)(C), §213(d)

8 Internal Revenue Code §162(a)

9 Internal Revenue Code §106(a), §105(b)

10 Treasury Regulations 1.105-5, 1.106-1

▼ N O T E S Premiums are considered qualifying medical expenses for purposes of the annual gift tax exclusion, if they are paid directly to the insurance carrier.[11]

Partnerships

Business partnerships can deduct eligible long-term care insurance premiums in a few different ways:

- The partnership can pay the entire premium and deduct it.[12]

- The premium is considered a *guaranteed payment* to a partner, is added to the partner's K-1 income and reported to the IRS on Forms K-1 and 1065.[13]

- A partner can deduct the eligible premium as a self-employment health insurance premium on Form 1040.[14]

- The partnership can deduct the actual premiums paid for other employees from business income. The premium is excluded from employee income, and benefits are tax-free.[15]

- The partnership can deduct the eligible premiums it paid for a partner's spouse and tax dependents, including parents.[16]

---

11 Internal Revenue Code §2503(e)

12 Internal Revenue Code §162(a)

13 Internal Revenue Code §61

14 Internal Revenue Code §162(1), 213(d)(1)(D)

15 Internal Revenue Code §106(a), §105(b)

16 Internal Revenue Code §162(l), §162(l)(2)(C), §213(d)

- The partnership can discriminate, offering the insurance to some employee classes, but not others.[17]

Example:

> Matthews & Fisher is a partnership. Sam Matthews, age 55, purchases a long-term care policy with a $2,000 annual premium. The eligible tax-deductible premium for his age is $1,020.
>
> Partner year-end K-1 distribution,
> before long-term care insurance premium $130,000
>
> Long-term care insurance premium $2,000
>
> K-1 income $132,000
>
> Eligible premium $1,110
>
> AGI less eligible premium $130,890

S corporations

Here are the various ways S corporations can deduct long-term care insurance premiums:

- The company can pay a shareholder's entire long-term care insurance premium and deduct it.[18] The premium is considered a *guaranteed payment* to a shareholder, is deemed part of the shareholder's salary, and is reported to him on form W-2, as well as to the IRS on the corporation's return, Form 1120S.[19]

---

17 Treasury Regulations 1.105-5, 1.106-1

18 Internal Revenue Code §162(a)

19 Internal Revenue Code §707(c)

- The shareholder can deduct the eligible premium as a *self-employment health insurance premium* on Form 1040.[20]

- The corporation can deduct the actual premiums paid for other employees from business income.[21] The premium is excluded from employee income, and benefits are tax-free.[22]

- The corporation can deduct the eligible premiums it paid for a shareholder's spouse and tax dependents, such as parents.[23]

- If a shareholder's domestic partner (heterosexual or same-sex) is a *bona fide* employee of the corporation, the shareholder can purchase a joint policy (naming one partner as owner and insuring both) and deduct the entire premium.[24] This opportunity is not available to lawful spouses, however.

- The corporation can discriminate, offering the insurance to some employee classes, but not others.[25]

Limited-liability companies (LLC)

An LLC is a form of legal protection for unincorporated individuals. It does not have its own tax status. LLCs owned by sole proprietors file as sole proprietorships (see page 132). LLCs with multiple owners usually file as partnerships (see page 133).

---

20 Internal Revenue Code §162(1), 213(d)(1)(D), §213(d)(10)

21 Internal Revenue Code §162(a)

22 Internal Revenue Code §106(a), §105(b)

23 Internal Revenue Code §162(l), §162(l)(2)(C), §213(d)

24 IRS Revenue Ruling 71-588

25 Treasury Regulations 1.105-5, 1.106-1

Professional corporations (PC)

Professional corporations can generally choose to be treated as C corporations (see page 137) or S corporations (see page 135); check with your state.

C corporations

Tax deductibility of long-term care insurance premiums is less restrictive for C corporations:

- The corporation can deduct the entire premium paid for an employee, regardless of whether he is also its shareholder.[26] The premium is excluded from the employee's income.[27]

- The corporation can deduct the entire premium it paid for a shareholder's spouse and tax dependents, such as parents.[28]

- Premium paid for a shareholder who is not an employee is not tax-deductible to the company.

- If a company shareholder does not claim his parents as tax dependents, he can have the company employ them, pay for their long-term care insurance and deduct the premiums.

- The corporation can discriminate, offering the insurance to some employee classes, but not others.[29]

---

26 Internal Revenue Code §162(a)

27 Internal Revenue Code §106(a), §105(b)

28 Internal Revenue Code §162(l), §162(l)(2)(C) and §213(d)

29 Treasury Regulations 1.105-5, 1.106-1

▼ N O T E S **State tax incentives**

Check the table on page 191 to determine whether your state offers any incentives to purchase long-term care insurance. Note, however, that these regulations do change, so check with your state for current information.

Employer-sponsored policies

There are three basic types of group policies: *true, affinity* and *multi-life.*

True group

In *true group insurance,* all members of the group are eligible for coverage, regardless of their health. For this reason, such policies' benefits tend to be more limited.

Although true group policies appear to be less expensive, they can lack options that may be appropriate for individual policyholders. The insured does not receive an individual policy, but a certificate of insurance signifying he or she is a member of a group plan.

Affinity group

Affinity insurance is made available by insurers through agreements with various organizations, such as teachers' unions or state bar associations. These are individual policies that may offer simplified underwriting for employees under a certain age. For example, an insurance company may underwrite individual purchasers under age 50 by asking a series of short questions in a phone interview. For older purchasers, the company requires an attending physician's statement. For affinity group insurance, the company may extend the simplified underwriting to purchasers up to a later age. In some cases, the employer contributes to the cost of the policy.

Multi-life

This is a term used by the long-term care insurance industry to denote groups covering small businesses (usually with fewer than 100 employees). The policies issued are generally the same as those offered to affinity groups.

Federal Long-Term Care Insurance Program

In 2002, the federal government entered into a marketing arrangement with MetLife and John Hancock Life Insurance (two long-term care insurance pioneers) to offer long-term care insurance to federal employees and their families, as well as active and retired military personnel. The resulting Federal Long Term Care Insurance Program (FLTCIP) is run by a firm established by the two insurers, Long-Term Care Partners, LLC.

FLTCIP policies are simple to understand and offer benefits tailored to their targeted audience. Policies are sold directly through highly trained, non-commission-based staff that understand how long-term care insurance works and how to recommend the right coverage.

Federal employees and their families are strongly advised to investigate this program.[30]

---

30 http://www.ltcfeds.com
http://www.opm.gov/insure/ltc/index.asp

▼ N O T E S **Long-Term Care Partnership programs**

Long-Term Care Partnership programs attempt to bring together the two major players in long-term care financing: the public sector, represented by state governments, and the private sector, represented by long-term care insurers. These cooperative efforts intend to make long-term care insurance more valuable to consumers by offering asset protection. Through these programs, owners of approved long-term care policies may qualify for Medicaid (see page 82), yet still protect their assets, even after their long-term care insurance benefits run out.

In 2006, Partnership programs were limited to California, Connecticut, Indiana and New York. Massachusetts has a variation of the concept. However, the Deficit Reduction Act of 2005 (DRA '05), signed into law by President George W. Bush on February 8th, 2006, paves the way for all states to create Partnership programs if they choose, and at least 20 states are considering doing so.

Current protection methods

Here is how the states that currently have Partnership programs treat assets, as of April 2007:

California and Connecticut: dollar-for-dollar asset protection

The plans in California and Connecticut permit dollar-for-dollar protection of assets for benefits purchased in a Partnership-approved long-term care policy. When you purchase a benefit pool in a particular amount, you can protect that amount from Medicaid (called Medi-Cal in California). Connecticut requires skilled nursing facilities and assisted-living facilities accepting Partnership policy reimbursement to offer a discount of 5% off the published daily room rate.

New York: unlimited asset protection

New York also offers dollar-for-dollar asset-protection policies, as well as policies with total (unlimited) asset protection. The latter permit the policyholder to qualify for Medicaid, once his long-term care benefits have been exhausted, without needing to spend down any of his assets. The state requires the purchase of a set minimum amount of long-term care benefits in order to protect assets.[31]

Indiana: hybrid asset protection

Indiana uses a hybrid model: the holder of a qualified long-term care policy with a pool of benefits below $217,186 (in 2007) protects his assets only in the amount of the policy's pool of benefits. However, if the consumer purchases benefits of just one dollar over $217,186, he protects unlimited assets.[32]

Massachusetts: selective asset protection

Massachusetts is not, formally, a Partnership state, but it does protect some assets in a similar way. The state will not place a lien on a home if the homeowner has a long-term care insurance policy with minimum daily coverage of $125 paying for at least two years of nursing-home care. Currently, the statute appears to offer protection only if the insured is in a nursing home, and not if he is receiving care at home or in an assisted-living facility.

Partnership programs: advantages and disadvantages

Partnership programs are attractive to consumers who might otherwise not have considered buying long-term care cover-

31 http://www.nyspltc.org/expansion.htm

32 http://www.in.gov/fssa/iltcp/state_set_chart.htm

▼ NOTES age. Once in place, these programs provide peace of mind to policy owners on two counts: they ensure that assets are protected to the extent of the benefits, and also that, if Medicaid is needed after all, it will be provided without most of the rigmarole that usually accompanies qualification.

There are two drawbacks, however:

- None of the Partnership programs protect individuals' incomes. If a policy owner is married and has substantial monthly income, a longer benefit period is strongly recommended. Going on Medicaid makes no sense because the income would go to the nursing home, placing the community spouse in financial jeopardy.

- The second drawback has to do with inflation protection. Most states mandate compound inflation in later years. The problem is that compound inflation protection usually doubles the cost of the policy. If cost is a serious concern, a non-Partnership policy that allows the policy owner to switch to simple inflation protection at an earlier age may be a more economical option.

Paying for a long-term care policy

The average long-term care insurance policy costs approximately $1,500 per year. Of course, the price increases with the insured's age at time of purchase and with the selection of any optional benefits. You may not wish to tap into your savings accounts each year to pay the premium. This section offers ideas on how to access the money to pay for a long-term care insurance policy.

Funding from an IRA

Many financial advisors have told me that few clients wish to draw down their IRAs starting at the mandatory age of 70½. Here's a suggestion: Instead of fully funding your IRA, consider diverting money starting in your early sixties to fund the premium on your long-term care insurance policy.

Example:

- Fred, who is 60 years old, opts for a 10-pay policy that provides him with a $150 daily benefit and a four-year benefit period, creating a $219,000 pool of funds. The premium for this policy is $3,500 a year.

- Instead of fully funding his IRA, he pays the premium with $2,000 that had been earmarked for the IRA and adds another $1,500 in cash.

- He will have to start drawing down his IRA at age 70½. The lost principal and interest on an annual investment of $2,000 for 10 years, accruing at 5%, is $29,671.

- The $219,000 pool of funds provided by the insurance far out paces the investment loss.

Reverse mortgages (Home Equity Conversion Mortgages, HECMs)

It's difficult to pick up a newspaper or magazine these days without reading about reverse mortgages. However, many consumers and professionals are not fully informed about their capabilities. Here is a crash course:

The formal name for reverse mortgages is *Home Equity Conversion Mortgages (HECMs)*. HECMs were created and are ad-

143

▼ N O T E S   ministered by the federal Department of Housing and Urban Development (HUD).

The lender agrees to advance a sum of money, either in a lump sum or on a periodic basis. The loan is secured with a mortgage on the borrower's house. Unlike a home-equity loan or refinancing, the interest accrues during the life of the borrower; no payment of either interest or principal is due until the owner dies, or sells or refinances the house. There is a maximum amount that can be borrowed, based on the home's location and other criteria.

To qualify, the homeowner must:

- be over 62;

- have a single-use dwelling such as a home, condominium or townhouse that meets Federal Housing Administration (FHA) guidelines;

- purchase insurance to cover any exposure that the lending institution may have, because the accrued balance may exceed the value of the house. The insurance guarantees that the heirs of the borrower will not be liable for any shortfall.

The money available is tax-free and does not count as income for Social Security eligibility purposes. The funds can be taken in several ways:

- Monthly payments over a period of years.

- A line of credit to be drawn on as needed.

- A combination of monthly payments and line of credit.

Some long-term care insurance advisors recommend that their clients pay for long-term care insurance with income from a reverse mortgage. It makes a lot of sense.

Life settlements

A life settlement is the assignment of a life insurance owner's death benefit in exchange for a lump sum payout now. The older and less healthy the owner is, the more cash he receives for the policy. Generally, to qualify for a life settlement, a person must:

- have a life expectancy of 12 years or less;

- be over 55;

- own a life-insurance policy with a cash surrender value and a face value of at least $100,000.

This type of transaction may be useful in these circumstances:

- The life insurance policyholder can no longer afford the premium or is about to let the life policy lapse and simply take the accumulated cash that has built over the years.

- The cash generated can fund a long-term care insurance policy or reduce debt.

- A business owner approaching retirement no longer needs a policy (in the cases of key-person policies or buy/sell coverage.)

Children contributing to the cost

This option is self-explanatory. It is often difficult for a parent to ask for assistance, so here is a suggestion: If there is a child who is more likely to provide care, the other children should contribute to the cost of the policy. The caregiver pays nothing—the care he or she gives is contribution enough. This can be a good way to help keep families together should a parent need extended care.

Buying the Right Long-Term Care Insurance Policy

7

When should you buy a long-term care insurance policy? 149

Step 1: Choosing the type of policy 150

    Individual 151

    Joint policy 151

    Linked policy 151

    Life insurance with an accelerated benefit 152

Step 2: Choosing a daily benefit amount 152

Step 3: Choosing a benefit period 153

    If cost is an issue 154

    If cost is not an issue 154

    If there's a history of longevity or chronic illness in your family 154

    If you have a portfolio that is heavy in tax-qualified or low-cost-basis assets 154

Step 4: Choosing an elimination period 155

    Days of service 155

    Calendar 156

    Hybrid 156

    Combination 157

Step 5: Choosing inflation protection 157

    Compound inflation protection 158

        When should you consider compound inflation protection? 159

    Simple inflation protection 160

        When should you consider simple inflation protection? 160

    No inflation protection at all 161

        When should you consider not buying inflation protection? 161

    Guaranteed option to purchase inflation protection in the future 161

    Inflation protection variations 162

    Can I do without inflation protection? 162

Step 6: Choosing how the policy pays the benefit 163

147

Reimbursement 163

Indemnity 164

Cash benefit 165

Step 7: Choosing a benefit payout schedule 166

Daily payout: unused daily benefit is not transferable 167

Weekly payout: unused daily benefit is transferable to other days in the same week 168

Monthly payout: maximizes flexibility 168

Additional options 169

Survivorship option 169

Accelerated-payment (limited-pay, paid-up) option 169

Nonforfeiture 170

Return-of-premium option 170

In my years of practice, I have seen more than a few poorly thought out long-term care insurance policies. I was left with the impression that the intent of the salesperson was to make a sale, not to help a family. The most egregious example is selling a $50 daily benefit in my state, Massachusetts, where the cost of nursing home care can run up to $270 per day.

Although the policy may have helped with some home care, it was worthless to protect income and assets when its insured was forced to apply for Medicaid. Ironically, the policy ended up helping not the family, but the state: once the insured was on Medicaid, the daily benefit was used to reduce what the state paid the facility.

The step-by step approach in this chapter will assist you in constructing the right long-term care policy for you. We strongly suggest that you work with a long-term care professional. For ideas on how to choose one, see page 179.

When should you buy a long-term care insurance policy?

Those who train long-term care insurance agents and brokers frequently advise them to suggest to consumers that the need for long-term care can happen at any age — just look at what happened to Christopher Reeves. What is often unsaid is that younger people have tremendous financial obligations and only limited funds to pay for insurance. When they do, they're better off investing in life and disability insurance.

The ideal time to consider purchasing the product is in your late fourties to early sixties for the following reasons:

- You are more likely to have had a direct experience with long-term care or to know a friend who is going through it.

- The need for insurance becomes more evident as you begin to see your friends get ill or perhaps die.

- In your late fifties, your retirement plans begin to gel and perhaps you can see how a long-term illness can have a devastating impact on them.

- Long-term care insurance is properly funded from income, not assets. Reallocating income to pay for care will likely have serious consequences to your lifestyle and, if the illness lasts long enough, to your surviving spouse or children who rely on your assets.

You can take a chance and wait until your late sixties or older to purchase long-term care insurance, but understand that insurance companies have substantially tightened their underwriting requirements. It is, simply, too risky to wait.

Step 1: Choosing the type of policy

The first step is to choose the right policy structure. There are four basic types:

1. *Individual*

2. *Joint*

3. *Linked* or *asset-based*

4. *Life insurance with an accelerated benefit*

Individual

As the name suggests, a policy of this type is structured to offer benefits to only one person. It can pay benefits the traditional way through a pool of benefits, or those benefits can be funded with the death benefits of a linked policy (see below).

Joint policy

This is one policy with, usually, one owner and two or more insured persons, including the owner. There are two advantages to this structure:

1. Even if one of the insured individuals does not use the policy, the benefits remain for the other(s).

2. Such policies are available at substantial discounts from the price of the appropriate number of individual policies.

Linked policy

This is not a stand-alone long-term care policy; rather, it is a rider on a traditional whole-life or universal-life insurance policy. The long-term care benefits are paid from the death benefit. Other than in its source of funding, a policy of this type is identical to an individual policy. The policy can pay one of two ways:

1. A monthly percentage of the death benefit

2. A monthly payment determined by dividing the death benefit by a number of months provided in the contract (usually 24, 36 or 48)

The obvious advantage of this structure is that the insured receives the face value of the policy one way or the other.

151

However, because the underwriting for the two types of insurance is opposite (mortality for the life insurance, morbidity for the long-term care insurance), the death benefit at the same premium is likely to be smaller than in a stand-alone life-insurance policy.

Life insurance with an accelerated benefit

Unlike a linked policy, a life policy with an accelerated benefit does not contain a long-term care insurance rider. Rather, it permits the policyholder to *accelerate* the death benefit—receive part or all of it while still alive—by drawing it down to pay for long-term care. One insurance company offers a rider that allows the policyholder to exceed the death benefit in paying for long-term care.

Step 2: Choosing a daily benefit amount

Once you've decided which type of policy is best for you, the next step is to determine your benefit amount—how much money per day the policy will pay toward your care.

Choosing a daily benefit amount requires a stepped approach:

1. Start by determining the highest cost of care in your community. This is probably the cost of nursing home care.

2. Add up your estimated annual expenses. Factor in, if you consider them important, any continuing post-retirement obligations you may have to your church, community, children or grandchildren.

3. Calculate your anticipated annual retirement income, including income from investments, even though you will most likely roll it over.

4. Subtract your annual expenses from your retirement income.

5. The difference is generally considered to be the amount you can use to contribute toward the cost of your care. It's called *coinsurance*.

6. From the highest cost of care in your area, subtract your coinsurance. The difference is the amount you should consider as a daily benefit.

Example:

> The most expensive nursing home in the town where David lives costs $75,000 per year. He estimates that he can comfortably spend $5,000 per year for his own care.
>
> Nursing home expense: $75,000
>
> Coinsurance: $5,000
>
> Yearly benefit needed: $70,000
>
> Daily benefit ($70,000 / 365): $190

Step 3: Choosing a benefit period

The next step is to determine how long your policy should pay benefits. Insurance companies have compiled some interesting statistics on how *long* long-term care actually is. Most of them report that their average claim is just under three years. Consider those statistics together with your family medical history and the financial consequences of guessing wrong.

The following recommendations are based on the purchase of a reimbursement policy, because it is the most common type

153

▼ NOTES of payment option. Benefit periods should be adjusted upward if you choose indemnity or cash-benefit payment (see the explanation of payment models starting on page 118).

Here are some suggestions based on financial and family considerations:

If cost is an issue

A three-year or four-year reimbursement benefit makes sense. The average claim lasts around three years. The reimbursement payment model stretches the actual time during which the policy pays with every day on which care costs less than the maximum daily benefit.

If cost is not an issue

Consider a longer benefit period, such as five or six years. This gives you an extra cushion.

If there's a history of longevity or chronic illness in your family

A lifetime benefit period is available, but its cost may be an issue.

If you have a portfolio that is heavy in tax-qualified or low-cost-basis assets

If you are in this category, you probably have a sophisticated plan for limiting taxes. Paying for care may mean liquidating qualified or low-cost-basis assets, resulting in an immediate tax liability. A lifetime benefit makes the most sense.

Step 4: Choosing an elimination period

One of the most confusing aspects of a long-term care insurance policy is the elimination period (see page 123). This is the period of time you have to wait between submitting a claim and receiving benefits. The period is anywhere from zero (the benefit is paid immediately upon submission of the claim) to one year. Also important is how the insurer counts the period.

Each insurer uses one of three methods to *run,* or count, an elimination period: *days of service, calendar,* and *hybrid.*

Days of service

A *days of service* elimination period is not counted in consecutive days like a calendar period. Instead, an elimination day is counted only if the policyholder receives at least one *compensable service* (a service for which the policy will pay) that day.

Example:

> If you choose a 60–day days-of-service elimination period and receive a home-care visit every other day, you will have to wait 120 days before benefits start. Generally, no credit is given for care provided by the insured's family or hospital stays.

Recommendation:

If cost is not an issue, choose a zero-day period but, in any case, no more than a 30-day days-of-service elimination period. Elimination periods are confusing, and when you or a loved one needs care, no-one might remember how this method works, especially in the likely event that the person filing the claim is not the policyholder.

▼ N O T E S **Calendar**

A *calendar* elimination period is the best method, but costs more. The policyholder does not need to show any paid care during the period.

A *calendar* elimination period is counted as consecutive days from the first claim for benefits, and not according to care actually given. No evidence of care need be shown to the insurer. Clearly, this is the best option, but it also costs more.

Example:

> Jules owns a policy with a 60-day calendar elimination period. He files the first claim on June 1st. His benefits will begin 60 consecutive days later, on July 31st. It doesn't matter whether he received care at any point between the initial claim and the end of the elimination period.

Recommendation:

If you want a longer elimination period, consider a 60-day calendar period. Your benefits will begin exactly 60 days after you filed the claim.

Hybrid

Many insurance companies offer the option of speeding up the elimination period by allowing you to claim seven days toward the elimination period whenever any care is received during a week, even if it is only on one day.

Example:

> Richard purchases a policy with a 90-day hybrid elimination period. After submitting his first claim for benefits, he shows one compensable service per day

each week for eight weeks. By doing so, he satisfies 56 days of his 90-day elimination period.

However, if you need more than one day of care per week, this will not speed up your elimination period any more.

Combination

Some insurers offer combination options, of which the most popular is a zero elimination period for home care and a 90-day elimination period for assisted-living or nursing-home care.

Recommendation:

The hybrid model may make sense if you are able to keep track of the days of the elimination period. I think it makes sense simply to select a shorter elimination period, or go with the combination option, particularly since it is likely that the initial care you may need would be at home.

Step 5: Choosing inflation protection

The cost of long-term care is likely to continue rising. To address this issue, insurance companies offer inflation protection, intended to keep daily benefit amounts rising as well. Depending on the policyholder's age, this option may be an essential part of the plan for long-term care.

Three basic types of inflation protection are offered, with several variations: *compound, simple* and an option that provides no current inflation protection but allows you to buy it in the future.

▼ NOTES **Compound inflation protection**

Compounding means that each year the increase in your daily benefit is calculated not on the original amount, but on the increased amount of the previous year. The inflation factor by which the previous year's daily benefit is increased each year is typically 5%.

Example:

- James purchases a $100 daily benefit with 5% compound inflation.

- In the policy's second year, the policy will pay 5% more than the original daily benefit: $105.

- In the third year, the daily benefit is 5% higher than it was in the second year: $110.25.

- In the fourth year, the daily benefit is 5% higher than it was in the third year: $115.76; and so on.

All carriers continue to compound the pool of funds even when the policy is paying benefits. However, the amount compounded is reduced as you draw down benefits.

Here's an example:

- Paul claims benefits for the first time in 2020. By then, his policy's compound inflation protection has increased his pool of benefits to $300,000.

- In his first year of receiving benefits, Paul draws the pool down by $25,000. This depletes his pool to $275,000 by the policy anniversary, and the insurer then compounds on that base value. The 5% compounding raises the pool to 288,750.

- In the second year of receiving benefits, Paul draws the NOTES▼ pool down by $40,000, to $248,750. The insurer compounds 5% on that base value, to $261,187.50; and so forth.

One insurer, however, continues to compound on the pool of funds that existed on the date the first claim for benefits was filed: payment of benefits does not reduce that amount.

Example:

- Michael claims benefits for the first time in 2020. By then, his policy's compound inflation protection has increased his pool of benefits to $300,000.

- In his first year of receiving benefits, Michael draws the pool down by $25,000. This depletes his pool to $275,000 by the compounding date. However, insurer compounds on the base value that existed on the date of the first claim. The 5% compounding raises the pool to 315,000; and so forth.

Always check with your long-term care professional to determine which benefit is best suited to you and your family's situation.

When should you consider compound inflation protection?

If you are under age 65 when you buy the long-term care insurance policy, consider compound inflation protection. You will probably not need care for many years. The benefit amount you select today may seem sufficient, but in twenty years, it may not be enough to cover the rising cost of care.

159

▼ N O T E S   **Simple inflation protection**

With this type of inflation protection, the original daily benefit amount increases by a set percentage (usually 5%) every year.

Example:

- In 2007, Stephen purchases a $100 daily benefit with 5% simple inflation protection. On every policy anniversary, his daily benefit amount will increase by 5% of the original benefit amount of $100, which equals $5.

- In the policy's second year, the daily benefit will be $105.

- In the policy's second year, the daily benefit will be $110; and so forth.

- The pool of benefits will also increase at the original 5% every year on the anniversary.

When should you consider simple inflation protection?

If you are between 65 and 75 years old, simple inflation protection is probably a better inflation option, since it costs less than compound and is likely to be almost as useful. The average first claim is generally filed around age 82. Because compound inflation protection doesn't increase the benefit substantially more than simple inflation until after 12 to 14 years, buying compound inflation protection at or after age 65 may not justify the cost.

No inflation protection at all

When should you consider not buying inflation protection?

If you are over 75, an inflation protection feature may not be worth the additional premium. As the average first claim is filed in one's eighties, it makes more sense to drop inflation protection altogether and buy a higher daily benefit. This will usually cost less and will initially give you a higher daily benefit, which may be useful if you need the policy relatively shortly after purchase.

Guaranteed option to purchase inflation protection in the future

Another inflation protection mechanism you can apply to your policy is a guaranteed option to purchase protection in the future. This allows you to keep the cost of your policy down, but reserves your right to increase your daily benefit amount in the future. However, you may not be able to increase you coverage once you become sick or disabled and are collecting benefits from your policy.

This is usually not a good choice for two reasons:

- If you don't exercise the option after a certain number of years, you generally lose the right to do so.

- If you do exercise the option, the premium for the inflation protection is based on your age at the time you do so, not when you first bought the policy. This could make the premium extremely expensive.

▼ NOTES **Inflation protection variations**

- Inflation tied not to a set rate (usually 5%) but to the Consumer Price Index (CPI). The thinking is that the cost of care has not outpaced the CPI for years. The premium is correspondingly lower on this feature.

- Double and out. The policy uses compounding to double the benefit and then stops. This may be a good idea if you are in your late sixties.

- Additional daily benefit purchase option. Traditional compounding continues unless you rewrite the policy to exclude it. One insurer automatically increases the daily benefit 5% per year but gives you the option of stopping the compounding benefit and restarting it.

Can I do without inflation protection?

In most cases, this is not a good idea. However, there are instances where opting not to protect against inflation is viable:

- You're 75 or older. A person in this age bracket is usually very close to using his long-term care insurance; he doesn't have many years for the inflation protection to increase the daily benefit amount. Ultimately, it's less expensive for him to buy a larger daily benefit than an inflation protection option.

- You're between 65 and 75 and you need to keep premiums down. In this situation, I would forego inflation protection and buy a higher daily benefit instead.

Step 6: Choosing how the policy pays the benefit

As you learned on page 118, your policy can pay benefits in one of three ways: *reimbursement, indemnity* or *cash.* Here's how each of these options works:

Reimbursement

Under the reimbursement model, the policyholder must submit bills to the insurance company for care that is covered in the insurance contract. The insurance company then reimburses either the owner of the long-term care insurance policy or the care provider.

Example:

> Jane purchases a $125 daily benefit, but needs only home care for two hours a day at a cost of $20 per hour. The insurer will either reimburse her for those $40, or pay the provider directly.

Advantage:

- This is the least expensive payment option because the daily benefit is unlikely to be drawn in full until the insured moves to a nursing home, and perhaps not even then. Whenever the daily benefit is not drawn in full, the balance becomes available for use on other days, effectively prolonging the benefit period.

  Example:

  > Bill purchases a $100 daily benefit with a four-year benefit period. However, he uses only $50 per day during this period, using up only half

his pool of benefits. His benefit period is thus effectively doubled.

Disadvantage:

- The policyholder receives benefits only to the extent of the actual cost of care. The policy is unlikely to pay for informal care, provided by family or friends, or alternative services such as holistic treatment.

Indemnity

An indemnity policy pays out the entire daily benefit, regardless of actual expenses, for any day on which at least one *compensable service* (covered service) is shown to have been performed.

Example:

Tom purchases an indemnity-based policy with a daily benefit of $125. On a particular day, he needs two hours of home care, which costs $20 per hour. The insurer pays him $125—the entire benefit amount. Tom pays his home care provider $40, and keeps the balance.

Advantages:

- The balances retained after payment for compensable services could be used to pay family members who help provide care.

- Some insurers allow indemnity benefits to be paid in other countries.

- If the insured's spouse or domestic partner cannot qualify for coverage and needs care, the care can be paid for through the insured's policy. Here's how this would work:

- The insured must go on claim.

- The family now contracts with, for example, a home health care agency to deliver a minimum amount of care per day (usually two hours) on a permanent basis. (Some carriers will also pay for a meals-on-wheels delivery.)

- The insured has now satisfied the requirement for a compensable service per day.

- The insurance company now pays the maximum daily benefit, and the family nets the difference between that and the cost of the service. That net amount can be used to pay for care of the uninsurable spouse.

Disadvantages:

- An indemnity-based policy costs more than an equivalent reimbursement-based one.

- The benefit period is not stretched automatically whenever the daily cost of care is below the daily benefit. The policyholder can extend the benefit period only by saving the unused daily payout balances.

Cash benefit

Cash benefit policyholders receive the entire daily benefit amount every day from the date after the elimination period ends until the benefit period ends. They need only present a plan of care calling for services; no care has to be given.

Advantages:

- This is a good option for people who want maximum flexibility, since the money can be used for any purpose. This may include, for example, payment of an alimony obligation.

- If the insured's spouse or domestic partner cannot qualify for coverage and needs care, the care can be paid for through the insured's policy; see page 172. The difference between doing this with a cash-benefit policy and an indemnity-based one is that a cash-benefit policy does not require any evidence of care.

- It can help pay for travel costs if you live in a rural area where professional care is difficult to find.

- It can be used to pay for care that wouldn't otherwise be covered, like holistic methods (yoga, alternative healing, prayer).

Disadvantages:

- The benefit period is not stretched automatically whenever the daily cost of care is below the daily benefit. The policyholder can extend the benefit period only by saving the unused daily payout balances.

- The cost of a cash-benefit policy can be as much as 50% more than that of an equivalent reimbursement-based policy.

Step 7: Choosing a benefit payout schedule

The benefit payout schedule confuses many people. It can allow you to carry over unused daily benefits to days when your actual cost of care exceeds your daily benefit. You can usually choose a daily, weekly or monthly payout schedule.

We will use the following example, and see how payment is rendered under each type of schedule:

> Gail has a long-term care insurance policy with a $150 daily benefit. She needs home care, which costs $20 an hour, a few days a week. Here's her care schedule:
>
> Monday: ....3 hours
>
> Wednesday: ....3 hours
>
> Friday: ....10 hours

Daily payout: unused daily benefit is not transferable

A daily payout schedule limits the policyholder to his maximum daily benefit. If care exceeds that amount, he cannot cover it with benefit from a day where care was less than the daily benefit.

Example:

> Gail needs only three hours of care on Mondays and Wednesdays, so her care on each of those days costs $60. Since her daily benefit is $150, she is reimbursed $60 for each of those days. The remaining $90 per day stays in her pool of benefits for future care.
>
> But on Fridays, Gail needs 10 hours of care, at a cost of $200.
>
> Because her policy employs a daily payout schedule, it pays only the $150 maximum daily benefit, leaving Gail to cover the remaining $50 out-of-pocket. She cannot use any of the money from Monday or Wednesday.

▼ NOTES **Weekly payout: unused daily benefit is transferable to other days in the same week**

This capability is usually purchased as an additional rider, but some insurers build it into the base policy. The benefits of weekly-payout policies can be transferred to cover care on other days in the same week on which care costs exceeded the daily benefit amount.

> This type of payout schedule could solve Gail's problem. For each defined week, the insurer will pay up to 7 times the daily benefit. The payout can be allocated among the days of that week as necessary to cover all compensable care, including days on which the daily benefit was exceeded.

Monthly payout: maximizes flexibility

This is the most flexible form of payout. It may be purchased as an additional rider, but some insurers build it into the base policy.

The principle is analogous to the weekly payout schedule: On a monthly-payout policy, the insurer will pay for all the care given each month, up to a month's worth of daily benefit.

Example:

> Gail's policy pays a daily benefit of $150. Her aggregate daily benefit for the month is $4,500.

> Gail's care schedule calls for 16 hours of care a week at $20 per hour. That's a cost of $320 per week, and a total cost of $1,280 for the month.

> With a monthly payout schedule, Gail would submit her $1,280 in care expenses to the insurance company.

Since her aggregate daily benefit amount doesn't exceed her care costs for the month, the insurance company would reimburse her for the full $1,280 amount. Any daily benefit amount she didn't use that month would remain in her pool of funds.

Additional options

Survivorship option

This benefit applies to couples that purchase policies together. Typically, if the policy's premiums have been paid for a certain number years (usually ten), and one spouse dies, the surviving spouse's policy is considered *paid up* (paid in full) and requires no further payments. This can be an important feature if there is an appreciable age difference between the spouses.

Accelerated-payment (limited-pay, paid-up) option

Most insurers allow policyholders to pay for their policies in full over a set period of time. At the end of the period, no further payment is due and the insurer cannot raise the premium in the future. This option is known as *accelerated payment, limited-pay,* or *paid-up.*

Accelerated payment may be attractive to younger, higher-income people who can afford to pay for the policy in a shorter amount of time. Some states don't allow this option, or do but mandate a *nonforfeiture* benefit. This option makes sense for business owners. See page 126.

▼ NOTES ## Nonforfeiture

Nonforfeiture must be offered as an option to all purchasers of tax-qualified long-term care policies. If this option is selected, and the policyholder stops paying the policy premiums after three years, he can elect *paid-up* status for the policy. This means that the policy will remain in force with a reduced maximum benefit, equal to the amount of premiums paid into the policy.

This rider may be worth considering if you are concerned that you might not be able to afford the premium payments in the future. However, the persistency rate on long-term care policies is very high: policyholders typically continue paying their premiums as they come due.

Return-of-premium option

This option provides for a return of the premiums paid for a long-term care policy at the insured's death. The refund is typically reduced by any benefits that had been paid on the policy, but some companies will refund all premiums paid without deducting any paid benefits. The refund can be made payable to the insured's estate or named beneficiary. Return-of-premium options are quite expensive, often almost doubling a policy's premium. It might interest those concerned by the prospect of spending money on a premium but never using the benefits. However, because of its cost, few people actually purchase this feature.

I Don't Qualify for Long-Term Care Insurance. Now What?

8

Paying for an uninsured spouse 172

Long-term care annuity 173

Medically underwritten single-premium immediate annuity (SPIA) 174

▼ N O T E S Funding a long-term care plan with a traditional long-term care insurance policy isn't an option for those who either cannot meet tough underwriting standards or already need long-term care. Here are some alternatives:

Paying for an uninsured spouse

There is a way for couples to pay, through the policy of a covered spouse or domestic partner, for the care of a spouse or domestic partner who is too sick to qualify for long-term care coverage.

The spouse who is able to qualify can use an indemnity or cash-benefit policy to help pay for the sick spouse's care. Here's how it works:

- The spouse who can qualify (often the wife) purchases an indemnity or cash-benefit long-term care policy for herself. The daily benefit should be selected on the basis of the couple's financial circumstances and the cost of care in their community.

- If the policyholder needs long-term care services, her policy begins to pay. The indemnity benefits allows her to get the entire daily benefit after she shows she has received at least one compensable service.

- The portion of the daily benefit remaining after payment for the policyholder's own care can be spent on needs not covered by the policy, including care for the spouse who is unable to qualify for his own policy.

- An indemnity policy is the more economical way to achieve this. A cash-benefit policy would work as well, but would cost more.

Long-term care annuity

An *annuity* is a contract between an insurance company and a client, called an *annuitant*. This contract states that the money he pays to the insurer will be repaid sometime in the future. A person whose health problems disqualify him from traditional long-term insurance may be able to qualify for a *long-term care annuity*.

This type of annuity allows the individual to purchase a long-term care insurance policy that usually has a benefit pool equal to the annuity purchased. The underwriting is greatly simplified because the annuity owner is required to use the annuity first to pay any long-term care expenses. The insurer starts paying benefits when the annuity is exhausted.

Example:

- Robert commits $100,000 to a deferred annuity. The carrier agrees to pay him an annual return of 4%. Robert also agrees not to draw any funds for a period of several years (usually 3 to 6 years).

- Robert now has the right to purchase long-term care insurance coverage with a benefit pool of $100,000, for an annual fee. The medical underwriting (medical criteria for qualification) is greatly simplified because the insurer is not liable until Robert exhausts his annuity paying for long-term care expenses.

- If Robert needs care, he first uses the funds in the annuity, including the accumulated interest. Let's assume that, by this time, interest has increased the annuity to $125,000.

- When that amount is depleted, Robert has access to the long-term care insurance policy's $100,000 benefit pool, which has increased to the amount to which the annuity had grown before Robert's first claim, $125,000.

- One insurer sells an unlimited long-term care benefit for an additional premium. It can be a smart idea.

Because of the simplified underwriting, a long-term care annuity is a great option for someone who has already been diagnosed with an illness that would disqualify him from purchasing traditional long-term care insurance.

Medically underwritten single-premium immediate annuity (SPIA)

This is an annuity that promises to pay the annuitant a sum of money for the rest of his life.

The payout of a traditional annuity is based on the annuitant's age, not health. For example, if an annuitant is 65 when he purchases the annuity, the payout calculation will be based on the life expectancy of an average 65-year-old. The calculation does not factor in the annuitant's health, even if he suffers from an illness, such as cancer, that can reduce life expectancy.

A *medically underwritten single-premium immediate annuity (SPIA),* on the contrary, is based only on the severity of the annuitant's illness, and not average life expectancy at his age. The sicker the annuitant, the less money he has to invest to obtain a guaranteed monthly income for life.

Example:

An 80-year-old man with moderate Alzheimer's disease needs $3,000 a month to cover long-term care costs.

	Traditional annuity	Medically underwritten SPIA
Age and sex	Male, 80	Male, 80
Health	Moderate	Moderate
Alzheimer's	No	Yes
Desired monthly income	$3,000	$3,000
Income duration	Lifetime	Lifetime
Lump-sum premium	$255,000	$118,000
Savings		$137,890

As the table demonstrates, it is possible to buy lifetime care through a medically underwritten SPIA for almost half of the cost of a traditional, age-based annuity.

The disadvantage of this strategy is that repayment on an annuity ceases when the annuitant dies. If he dies sooner than the insurer expects, the insurer retains the portion of the premium that has not been repaid.

Some insurance companies offer the option of a refund of some of that principal when the annuity holder dies. The beneficiary would receive a reduced amount of the principal in monthly payments.

Choosing a Long-Term Care Professional

9

Agents *vs* brokers 178

How to find a long-term care insurance specialist 179

    Word of mouth 179

    The Internet 179

Questions to ask your long-term care insurance professional 180

    Training 180

    Professional designation 180

▼ NOTES Long-term care insurance is a complex product. While I hope this book has helped you understand what you should look for in a policy, I don't recommend making this purchase by yourself, or online. There are just too many variables to consider.

If you decide that long-term care insurance is the best way to fund your long-term care plan, please seek the assistance of a qualified professional. This person should have a big-picture perspective of what you're trying to accomplish. He or she should, first of all, have the capacity to help you create a plan that will protect your family. Only after that plan is established, should the conversation turn to designing a long-term care insurance policy that will fund your plan.

The following information will help you find a qualified, well-rounded long-term care insurance professional.

Agents *vs* brokers

The terms *agent* and *broker* are often misunderstood.

An agent works for a particular insurance company. This person can be expected to believe strongly in his company's products, and to feel that, on balance, they are the best-suited for the insurer's targeted market. The insurance company invests a great deal of money in the agent's training and professional support. In the past, agents were not allowed to recommend other insurers' products; however, that is not always true today.

A broker is an independent business person who represents many insurance companies. Brokers often say that because they are not beholden to a particular company, they can better recommend the right product for a particular situation. This may be true in some cases, but it's important to note that insurance companies sometimes offer brokers attractive incentives to promote their products.

While it's important to understand the manner in which long-term care insurance agents and brokers work, one is not necessarily better than the other. As you shop around for a professional, your focus should be on that person's competence, and not his business model.

How to find a long-term care insurance specialist

Word of mouth

It's likely that word-of-mouth is how you found your lawyer, physician, accountant, or other professionals. And these professionals may be able to recommend good long-term care insurance specialists. But before you do, ask for a referral from a professional you already work with, make sure he or she understands the main aspects of long-term care.

The Internet

Performing a Web search for a "long-term care insurance specialist" will help you locate people who say they understand long-term care, but it's important to do a little additional digging before you give them a call. Visit the professional's website and investigate his or her credentials.

A website with some wonderful tools to help you is ElderLaw-Answers.[1] This site was created by Harry Margolis, an elder-law attorney who strongly believes in planning for long-term care and protecting that plan with long-term care insurance.

---

1   http://www.ElderLawAnswers.com

▼ N O T E S It is a clearinghouse of information on attorneys, agents and brokers in the long-term care insurance business. The site includes a searchable database of elder-law attorneys by area code or city and state.

Questions to ask your long-term care insurance professional

Ronald Reagan once said: "Trust but verify." Hopefully the agent or broker you choose is being honest about his or her credentials. But just in case, you can make sure by asking some questions:

Training

- *"What kind of long-term care training have you had?"*

- *"Did the courses focus on selling long-term care insurance, or working with families to establish a plan for long-term care?"*

If the professional seems to indicate that the training focus was on selling the product, rather than the issues I've discussed in this book, he or she may lack the outlook and experience required to craft and fund a viable long-term care plan.

Professional designation

- *"Do you hold a professional long-term care designation?"*

- *"What is it?"*

There are four nationally recognized programs that offer designations for long-term care professionals. If the professional you're talking to has any of these, consider it a good sign that he or she has an understanding of the long-term care issues that can affect your family.

- Long-Term Care Professional (LTCP).[2] This designation is offered through the American Association for Long-Term Care Insurance (a trade group that promotes selling and marketing ideas to its members) and America's Health Insurance Plans (which represents health-care insurers).[3] This program emphasizes long-term care needs and options, financing those needs, long-term care insurance and the administration of insurance claims.

- Certified Senior Advisor (CSA).[4] This professional designation takes a holistic and spiritual look at the problems facing seniors and their families. It does not offer a comprehensive evaluation of proficiency in long-term care insurance.

- Certified in Long-Term Care (CLTC).[5] This is the long-term care insurance industry's only third-party professional program. It is not funded by any insurance company. The CLTC designation is owned by a nonprofit organization completely independent of the insurance industry. Courses focus on training professionals to assist clients in preparing a plan for long-term care and, if appropriate, recommend long-term care insurance to fund that plan.[6]

- Chartered Advisor for Senior Living (CASL).[7] The American College is a well-known and respected institution that offers a variety of insurance programs and

2 http://www.aaltci.org

3 http://www.ahip.org

4 http://www.csa.org

5 http://www.ltc-cltc.com

6 The author is the principal founder and creator of this designation.

7 http://www.theamericancollege.edu/advance/casl/default.asp?section=6

designations. Its CASL program focuses on the unique issues that mature clients face during retirement years. The American College has recently partnered with the CLTC program to offer its CASL designation to CLTC graduates.

Appendix: State Medicaid Worksheet

A

You should be familiar with the rules of your state's Medicaid program to understand how they affect Medicaid qualification, discussed starting on page 82. The following worksheet covers the most common state-specific information. Please call your local Medicaid office for the information.

Countable assets in your state

Assets deemed countable in most states

	Countable	Non-countable
Stocks	☐	☐
Bonds	☐	☐
Savings	☐	☐
Money-market accounts	☐	☐
CDs	☐	☐
Tax-qualified pension plans	☐	☐
Single-premium deferred annuity	☐	☐
Life Insurance with cash surrender value	☐	☐
Vacation property	☐	☐
Investment property	☐	☐

▼ N O T E S **Other assets deemed countable in your state**

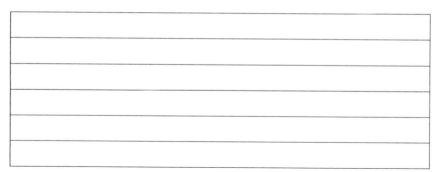

Circumstances under which tax-qualified pension plans will not be considered available to be spent on a Medicaid applicant's care

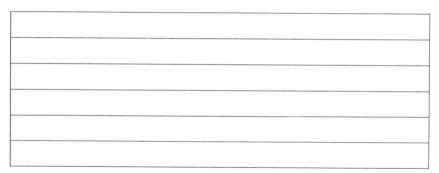

Types of life insurance deemed countable, and the criteria determining that status

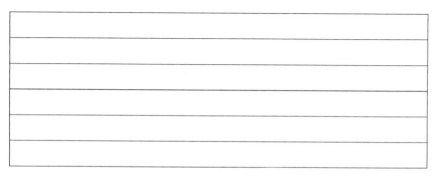

Non-countable assets in your state

Assets deemed non-countable in most states

	Countable	Non-countable
Car	☐	☐
Principal residence	☐	☐
Business supporting family	☐	☐
Business property	☐	☐
Household goods	☐	☐
Prepaid funeral	☐	☐
Burial account	☐	☐
Term life insurance	☐	☐ under $_____
Cash	☐	☐ under $_____

Other assets deemed non-countable in your state

▼ N O T E S **Primary residence**

Policy on placing liens on the primary residence

Income

Cap state

A cap state (see page 88) will not grant Medicaid eligibility to anyone whose income exceeds a cap. As of April 2007, the cap, adjusted annually, was $1,869, and the cap states were:

- Alabama
- Alaska
- Arizona
- Arkansas
- Colorado
- Delaware
- Florida
- Idaho
- Iowa
- Louisiana
- Mississippi
- Nevada
- New Mexico
- Oklahoma
- Oregon
- South Carolina
- South Dakota
- Texas
- Wyoming

Are you in a cap state?

☐ Yes; the cap is $_____   ☐ No

Income and asset rules for couples

Minimum monthly maintenance needs allowance (MMMNA)

Your state's MMMNA: $_____

Other expenses that may be added to the MMMNA

Community spouse resource allowance (CSRA)

Your state's CSRA: $_____

Appendix: Medicaid Life Expectancy Tables

B

Life expectancy of men

Age	To live	Age	To live	Age	To live	Age	To live	Age	To live
0	71.80	24	49.55	48	28.02	72	10.08	96	2.74
1	71.53	25	48.63	49	27.17	73	10.27	97	2.60
2	70.58	26	47.72	50	26.32	74	9.27	98	2.47
3	69.62	27	46.80	51	25.48	75	9.24	99	2.34
4	68.65	28	45.88	52	24.65	76	8.76	100	2.22
5	67.67	29	44.97	53	23.82	77	8.29	101	2.11
6	66.69	30	44.06	54	23.01	78	7.83	102	1.99
7	65.71	31	43.15	55	22.21	79	7.40	103	1.89
8	64.73	32	42.24	56	21.43	80	6.98	104	1.78
9	63.74	33	41.33	57	20.66	81	6.59	105	1.68
10	62.75	34	40.23	58	19.90	82	6.21	106	1.59
11	61.76	35	39.52	59	19.15	83	5.85	107	1.50
12	60.78	36	38.62	60	18.42	84	5.51	108	1.41
13	59.79	37	37.73	61	17.70	85	5.19	109	1.33
14	58.82	38	36.83	62	16.99	86	4.89	110	2.74
15	57.85	39	35.94	63	16.30	87	4.61	111	1.25
16	56.91	40	35.05	64	15.62	88	4.34	112	1.17
17	55.97	41	34.15	65	14.96	89	4.09	113	1.10
18	55.05	42	33.26	66	14.32	90	3.86	114	1.02
19	54.13	43	32.37	67	13.70	91	3.64	115	0.96
20	53.21	44	31.49	68	13.09	92	3.43	116	0.89
21	52.29	45	30.61	69	12.50	93	3.24	117	0.83
22	51.38	46	29.74	70	11.92	94	3.06	118	0.77
23	50.46	47	28.88	71	11.35	95	2.90	119	0.66

Life expectancy of women

Age	To live	Age	To live	Age	To live	Age	To live	Age	To live
0	78.79	24	55.95	48	33.17	72	13.99	96	3.16
1	78.42	25	54.98	49	32.27	73	13.33	97	2.97
2	77.48	26	54.02	50	31.37	74	12.68	98	2.80
3	76.51	27	53.05	51	30.48	75	12.05	99	2.64
4	75.54	28	52.08	52	29.60	76	11.43	100	2.48
5	74.56	29	51.12	53	28.72	77	10.83	101	2.34
6	73.57	30	50.15	54	27.86	78	10.24	102	2.20
7	72.59	31	49.19	55	27.00	79	9.67	103	2.06
8	71.60	32	48.23	56	26.15	80	9.11	104	1.93
9	70.61	33	47.27	57	25.31	81	8.58	105	1.81
10	69.62	34	46.31	58	24.48	82	8.06	106	1.69
11	68.63	35	45.35	59	23.67	83	7.56	107	1.58
12	67.64	36	44.40	60	22.86	84	7.08	108	1.48
13	66.65	37	43.45	61	22.06	85	6.63	109	1.38
14	65.67	38	42.50	62	21.27	86	6.20	110	1.28
15	64.68	39	41.55	63	20.49	87	5.79	111	1.19
16	63.71	40	40.61	64	19.72	88	5.41	112	1.10
17	62.74	41	39.66	65	18.96	89	5.05	113	1.02
18	61.77	42	38.72	66	18.21	90	4.71	114	0.96
19	60.80	43	37.78	67	17.48	91	4.40	115	0.89
20	59.83	44	36.85	68	16.76	92	4.11	116	0.83
21	58.86	45	35.92	69	16.04	93	3.84	117	0.77
22	57.89	46	35.00	70	15.35	94	3.59	118	0.71
23	56.92	47	34.08	71	14.66	95	3.36	119	0.66

Appendix: State Tax Incentives C

States that allow a deduction of all or a portion of the premium:

- Alabama
- Arizona
- Colorado
- Idaho
- Illinois
- Indiana
- Iowa
- Kentucky
- Maine
- Maryland
- Minnesota
- Missouri
- Montana
- New Hampshire
- New Jersey
- New Mexico
- Ohio
- Utah
- Virginia
- Wisconsin

States that allow a credit against taxes for all or a portion of the premium:

- New York
- North Carolina
- North Dakota
- Oregon

▼ NOTES

States that offer the same deductions as the federal government (deduction is based on the policyholder's age):

- Arkansas
- California
- Delaware
- Dist. of Columbia
- Georgia
- Hawaii
- Kansas
- Massachusetts
- Mississippi
- Nebraska
- Oklahoma
- Rhode Island
- South Carolina
- Vermont

States without tax incentives to purchase long-term care insurance:

- Connecticut
- Louisiana
- Michigan
- Pennsylvania

Index

A

Accelerated-payment option **126, 169**

Activities of daily living (ADLs)

     as long-term care insurance trigger **122**

     as Medicaid custodial-care eligibility trigger **82**

     definition **30**

Adult day care centers **33**

Advisors, choosing the right **179**

Alternate plan of care **124**

Annuities

     and Medicaid eligibility **101**

     Medically underwritten SPIA **174**

Assets, and Medicaid eligibility **83**

Assisted-living facilities **34**

B

Bed reservation **124**

Benefit tax deductibility **130**

Benefit triggers **122**

Business deduction of premiums

     C corporations **137**

     Limited-liability companies (LLC) **136**

     Partnerships **134**

     Professional corporations (PC) **137**

     S corporations **135**

     Self-employed individuals (sole proprietors) **132**

Buying the right policy

     Accelerated-payment (limited-pay, paid-up) option **169**

     Age at purchase **149**

     Benefit payout schedule: daily, weekly or monthly **166**

     Benefit period **153**

     Daily benefit **152**

193

Elimination period...**155**
Inflation protection **157**
Payment model: reimbursement, indemnity or cash benefit....................**163**
Return-of-premium option **170**
Survivorship option **169**
When to purchase **149**
Which type: individual, joint, etc...**150**

C

Cap states...**89**
Care coordination **124**
Care, levels of...**30**
Cash benefit..**165**
Choosing the right policy. *See Buying the right policy*
Cognitive impairment...**123**
Coinsurance **153**
Community spouse resource allowance (CSRA).......................**86**
Consumer Reports **110, 113, 114**
Continuing Care Retirement Communities............................**35**
Custodial care...**30**

D

Deductibility of long-term care insurance benefits **130**
Deductibility of long-term care insurance premiums...............**130**
Deficit Reduction Act of 2005.................**82, 84, 92, 101, 140**
Dialogue, starting one with your family about a plan...............**23**
Difference between Medicare and Medicaid.......................**61, 79**
Disabled child..**104**
Divorced or widowed individuals **46**

E

Elimination period **123**
Employer-sponsored insurance **138**

Estate recovery **101**

F

Federal Long-Term Care Insurance Program **139**

G

Gifts
    and Medicaid eligibility **85, 102**
    illegal under Medicaid state law **102**
Group long-term care insurance **138**
Guaranteed renewability **121**

H

Home care **16, 33**
    services covered by Medicaid **81**
Home equity, can disqualify from Medicaid benefits **93**
Home equity conversion mortgages (HECMs) **59**
Home equity loans **59**
Home-health-care-only policies **120**
Home modification **124**
Home, protecting a **104**
Hospitalization, requirement for prior
    prohibited in long-term care policies **121**

I

Income, and Medicaid eligibilityqualification **88**
Indemnity **164**
Inflation protection **157**

L

Lawyer, choosing a **105**
Levels of care **30**
Life estates, Medicai estate recovery against **99**

Limited-pay option **126, 169**

Long-term care

    consequences of **21**

    definition **15, 30**

    risk vs consequences **19**

Long-term care insurance

    history of...**115**

    How policies work **117**

    non-tax-qualified **129**

    policy language **121**

    tax-qualified **127**

Long-term care is rarely nursing-home care...**16**

Long-Term Care Partnership programs **140**

Look-back period **85**

M

Marriage

    Medicaid treatment of assets...**86**

    with children, developing a plan...**43**

    without children, developing a plan **42**

Medicaid..**79**

    coverage of home health care **81**

    covered services...**80**

    eligibility **82**

    planning **94**

    planning in a crisis..**103**

Medical necessity **123**

Medicare **61**

    coverage of nursing-home care..**63, 64**

Miller trusts, for Medicaid eligibility in cap states **89**

Minimum monthly maintenance needs allowance (MMMNA)...........................**90**

N

Nonforfeiture **126**

Nursing homes
    definition **36**
    Medicare coverage of... **63**

P

PACE, Program of All-Inclusive Care for the Elderly........................ **81**
Paid-up option **126, 169**
Partnership programs... **140**
Planning for long-term care
    Starting a dialogue about long-term care with your family........... **23**
    What is it? **22**
Premiums on long-term care insurance
    state tax incentives... **191**
    Tax deductibility of... **130**
Prenuptial agreements, not valid for Medicaid eligibility................... **87**

R

Reimbursement **163**
Residence, protecting a **104**
Respite care... **125**
Restoration of benefits **124**
Return-of-premium option **127, 170**
Reverse mortgages **59**

S

Same-sex couples, developing a plan **47**
Second marriage with children, developing a plan............................ **44**
Single
    with children, developing a plan... **40**
    without children, developing a plan..................................... **39**
Skilled care... **32**
Skilled nursing facilities.. **36**
Statistics on long-term care **16**

Supplemental-needs trusts (SNTs) for disabled children **104**
Survivorship option **125, 169**

T

Thirty-day free look **121**
Trusts **99**
    irrevocable **100**
    Miller Trusts, for Medicaid qualification in a cap state **89**
    revocable **100**
    supplemental-needs trusts (SNTs) for disabled children **104**

V

Veterans Administration
    benefits **69**
    payment for custodial care **70, 73**

W

Waiver of premium **125**